PELOTON HACKS

PELOTON HACKS

GETTING THE MOST FROM YOUR BIKE

An Unofficial Guide of More Than
100 Tips, Tricks, and Pieces of Advice

MARK A. GOMPERTZ

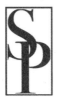

Skyhorse Publishing

Skyhorse Publishing books may be purchased in bulk at special discounts for sales promotion, corporate gifts, fund-raising, or educational purposes. Special editions can also be created to specifications. For details, contact the Special Sales Department, Skyhorse Publishing, 307 West 36th Street, 11th Floor, New York, NY 10018 or info@skyhorsepublishing.com.

Skyhorse® and Skyhorse Publishing® are registered trademarks of Skyhorse Publishing, Inc.®, a Delaware corporation.

Visit our website at www.skyhorsepublishing.com.

10 9 8 7 6 5 4 3 2 1

Library of Congress Cataloging-in-Publication Data is available on file.

Cover design by Brian Peterson

Print ISBN: 978-1-5107-6143-8
Ebook ISBN: 978-1-5107-6144-5

Printed in the United States of America

Always consult with your physician before beginning any new form of exercise program.

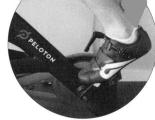

TABLE OF CONTENTS

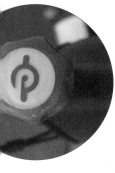

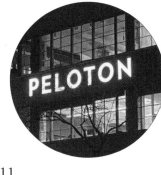

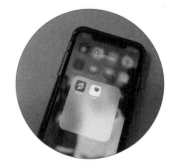

Part 4: USING THE TABLET

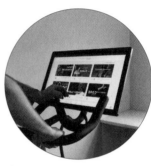

Part 5: MAKING THE MOST OF YOUR CLASSES

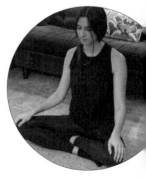

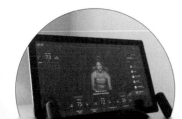

Part 6: PELOTON OUT IN THE WORLD

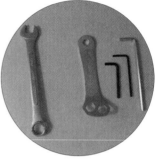

Part 7: THE INS AND OUTS OF YOUR BIKE

Part 8: SELF IMPROVEMENT . . . AND FUN!

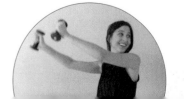

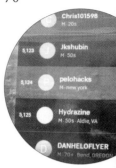

Part 9: CONNECTING TO OTHERS

Part 10: STRETCHING

Part 11: STRENGTH TRAINING AND YOGA

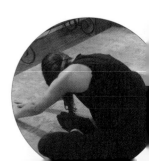

Part 12: OTHER WORKOUT OPTIONS

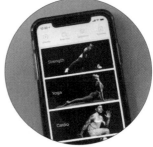

For Julian, Zachary, and Penny,
whose love motivates me to get on the bike every chance I get.

• •

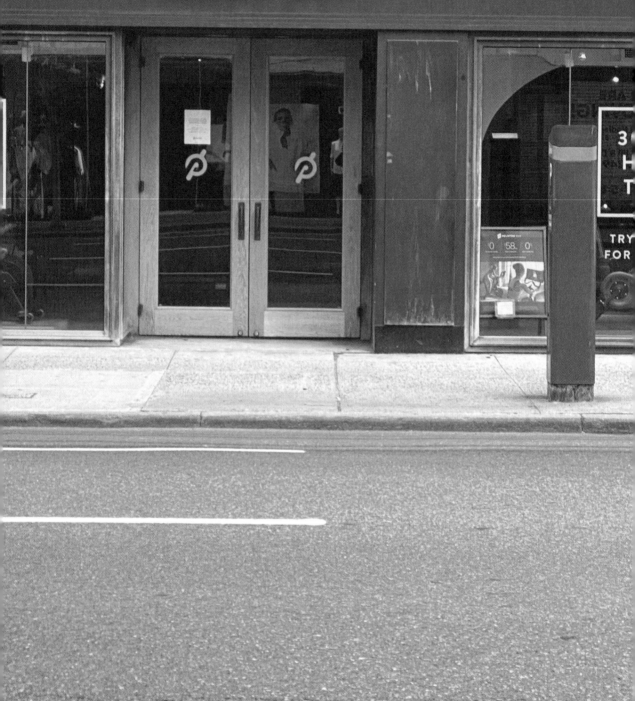

INTRODUCTION

On the day after Thanksgiving—which also happened to be my wedding anniversary—my wife and I were feeling particularly overstuffed and out of shape. A number of things can happen when you feel this way. You can get down on yourself. You can resolve to eat better in the future. You can avoid mirrors at all costs. But one of them is suddenly finding yourself at the Peloton store, which was precisely what happened to us.

The friendly sales representative asked how she could assist us.

"Deborah," I said, reading her name tag. "Take a good look at me."

She appeared momentarily confused as I continued.

"Do I look like someone in one of your commercials? I'm not young, and I'm not already in shape—with great muscle tone and a jaw like a quarterback. Why should someone at my age and with my build purchase your bike *and* subscribe to your streaming service of fitness classes? Frankly, it all seems daunting."

"We have a lot of great beginner and interval training programs," she replied without batting an eye. "Do you like Soul Cycle or Flywheel?"

"I hate working out in front of other people."

This seemed to be enough for her to render a diagnosis.

Deborah said, "Then the Peloton Bike is perfect for you. You'll have the benefit of those types of classes—group classes—but you'll have the flexibility to do the workouts in the privacy of your own home. Would you like to try the bike out here at the store?"

I was not dressed for a workout and had not planned on exercising that day. (And I was, as you will recall, still overstuffed from Thanksgiving.) Yet none of this was a problem. Deborah lent me a pair of special shoes, and before I could say Greg LeMond, I was clipped in and pedaling on a Peloton. After five minutes, I announced that "this isn't so hard after all."

"Uh . . . you're just in the warm-up stage," she pointed out.

I chose not to take this personally.

I looked over at my wife, who nodded in approval. She liked the workout and she liked the bike— so far, so good.

Then I asked about the price. Let's just say it was a good thing I was still clipped in . . . because otherwise I might have fallen off the bike. Peloton Bikes were—to say the least—not cheap.

But couples sometimes make "big purchases" if something is important or special. My wife immediately let me know that she saw a way that this could be both.

It would be the perfect anniversary gift, she told me. And it could be one we give each other.

"That's not very romantic," I replied.

"Are you kidding?" she asked. "What could be better to give each other than the gift of health? What could be more romantic than staying in shape for each other?"

The more I thought about it, the more I couldn't argue with it.

Deborah, it turned out, had seen this movie before. From across the Peloton store showroom, she flashed a knowing smile.

* * *

It is no secret that there are enormous health benefits to indoor cycling. It can reduce your overall body fat and help you drop pounds. When you ride a bike—stationary, outdoor, or otherwise—you're using some of the largest muscles in your body: the gluteus maximus and the quadriceps. "Spinning"—a.k.a. riding a stationary bike like a Peloton—can burn a tremendous number of calories. Some workouts will run you six hundred calories or more. An intense ride on a Peloton gives you an optimal cardio workout—increasing heart and lung capacity, while also toning your leg and butt muscles and getting rid of some of those excess pounds.

Some newer studies have also shown that spinning may trigger the release of chemicals that could lead to blood vessel repair and renewal.

So it's the complete package. An intense cycling workout can help improve body composition, decrease fat mass, and also lower your blood pressure and cholesterol.

Does this already sound too good to be true? Are you wondering if there are any drawbacks?

Well, there aren't any surprises, if that's what you mean. But it *is* possible to try to do too much, too quickly. As with any other form of exercise, overexertion—especially when you first begin the activity—can lead to injury. The good news is that, with a Peloton, you'll know when you're taking it to the limit. Your body will tell you. And the metrics on the bike will, too. It's also quite intuitive when it comes to easing yourself into a Peloton workout. Keep yourself hydrated properly and give your muscles time to adapt to the intensity of the workout.

When begun carefully and in moderation—at least at first—the type of vigorous aerobic exercise offered by a Peloton has very few risks and many potential benefits.

Bike-based exercise can be excellent for athletes at all levels who are beginning to suffer from joint issues that arise from higher-impact workouts (such as running).

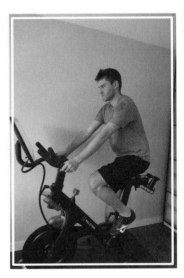

A high-intensity Peloton workout is good for mental health, as well. After a bike-based workout, you will feel your energy and mental focus improve, and you'll have more energy as you go through the rest of your day. Vigorous exercise releases endorphins, which tend to put people in a better mood and give them a pleasant sense of calm. In addition, scientists have found that after spinning, there is increased blood flow to the brain. The upshot is that it keeps you mentally sharper while improving your concentration, memory, reasoning, and planning. Again and again, studies by exercise physiologists find that spinning can elevate your mood, relieve anxiety, and reduce stress. And those are just the short-term benefits. Over the long term, we're finding that twenty to thirty minutes of riding a day can actually prevent depression.

And who are we to argue with science? With so much good data to recommend it, all the evidence makes a very strong case for the benefits of a Peloton workout.

What does the word *peloton* mean? As it turns out, the word derives from the French word for "little ball." In the military sense, it can be used to mean "platoon," but in a road bicycle race, like the Tour de France, "the peloton" is the word used to refer to a cluster or group of riders. A group of bikes together is a peloton.

The company that produces the Peloton exercise machine—Peloton Interactive—was founded in 2012, but it wasn't until 2014 that they started selling their namesake exercise bikes. Although numbers vary depending on which source you use—probably because there are discrepancies regarding how many people own the bikes, how many households have multiple users, how many people just use the app, and who uses the bike in a gym or hotel—hundreds of thousands of people are using Peloton today. Suffice it to say, it has grown tremendously since its origins and shows little sign of slowing down.

When the product was first introduced, many on Wall Street didn't believe Peloton Interactive would succeed because, the thinking went, "You can't be a hardware *and* a software company." And Peloton, of course, involves both the physical exercise bike and the creation and deployment of the visual content that complements the bike-riding experience. But this was one instance in which the Wall Streeters were proved wrong! Peloton's unique approach has paid off—with an emphasis on "paid"—because in addition to selling an expensive bike and touch screen tablet, the company makes a lot of money off the subscriptions it sells. At the time of this writing, Peloton Interactive is valued at an astonishing four billion dollars.

The headline of a recent *New York Times* article about Peloton Interactive read, "PELOTON IS A PHENOMENON. CAN IT LAST?" I'm not a betting man, but everyone I know who has tried a Peloton Bike loves it.

So I'd give it more than even money of lasting a good long time.

The popularity of Peloton Bikes is not hard to understand when you sit back and think about it. The product was introduced during a cultural and business cycle (no pun intended) that saw the rise of health and wellness activities. Coupled with a new focus on nutrition, more and more Americans are looking at ways to get healthier through exercise. Cycling has seen a particular boom in recent years. There's always been a baseline of people who like bike riding (both outdoors and indoors). This has been true since a French baby carriage mechanic first invented the modern bicycle! But what explains the newest boom? One answer is the rise of cycling fitness gyms like SoulCycle. SoulCycle has developed a devoted following—some have even called it "cult-like"—and many adherents describe it as a way of life! But the popularity of SoulCycle is not the full explanation. Indeed, if we look more closely, we can see that SoulCycle is more a symptom than a cause.

The answer, truly, is technology.

When we look at exercise trends over the decades—from aerobics to Tae Bo videotapes—we see that technology is always a driver. People everywhere are always looking for exercise that is accessible, engaging, and as tailored and customized as it can be. In the 1980s, for example, we saw the explosion of aerobics. Aerobics routines could be customized to the fitness level of those who participated, while "aerobics studios" offering group classes abounded. Consumers could also enjoy the convenience of doing aerobics in their own homes. Then-cutting-edge technology—the VCR—made this crucial aspect of the aerobics experience possible.

Through the end of the twentieth century and into the twenty-first, we've seen enhancements and refinement driven by other technological innovations such as the Internet, DVDs, wireless technology, and streaming.

With Wi-Fi devices nearly omnipresent, the time is now right for Peloton!

In addition to technology, another factor that I strongly believe has helped ensure the rise of Peloton is the increasing challenge of finding a "work/life balance" and making time for exercise activities. In blue-collar jobs, Americans are working longer and longer hours. And in white-collar ones, technology has made connection to "the office" near-to-constant, with workers pressured to address job projects during all their waking hours.

While American workers look for ways to address these challenging trends, they still need to find ways to sneak in a workout whenever they can!

This challenge of being time-strapped was crucial to the founding of Peloton, and that's not hyperbole. Consider the origin story of the founder, John Foley. He and his wife had always loved working out, and they enjoyed going to spin classes whenever they could find time. But with two small children at home, it was a constant challenge. It seemed they could never find the time to get to a studio.

But there is wisdom in the aphorism: "Necessity is the mother of invention."

Thus a company was born.

Peloton now has over eighty brick-and-mortar locations in the United States, Canada, the United Kingdom, and, more recently, Germany. And it shows no sign of stopping. The company plans to open many more stores in the next decade and is especially targeting high-end malls. On the content-creation side, the company is also growing and robust. It employs thirty-four full-time instructors who stream over twenty live classes per day. And Peloton's permanent library now offers thousands of on-demand classes, too.

So we know that Peloton is on the leading edge of exercise solutions that technology is making possible. We also know that it's an innovative, growing company that shows no signs of stopping. But is a Peloton the right piece of exercise equipment for you?

When thinking about whether or not you want one of these remarkable devices in your home, it's important to consider the quality of what you will be getting. The question is not only how well it will perform, but how well it is designed. There are several imitators and "knockoffs" of Peloton. But I hope I can convince you to go with the real thing.

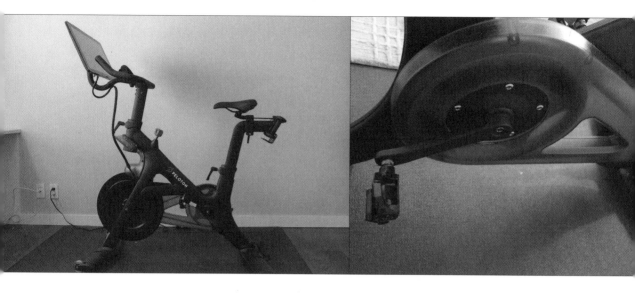

The Peloton Bikes are made of cutting-edge material like carbon steel and aluminum. From across the room, you can appreciate that this is something that's really designed and built to exacting specifications with the user in mind. (And I have to add—to put it in layman's terms—this means they're really cool-looking, and a great conversation piece!)

Peloton Bikes have a weighted flywheel in the front that provides electromagnetic resistance that the user can adjust. The feels-larger-than-it-is, twenty-two-inch touch screen attached to the front of the bike runs streaming content in high definition. That content consists of a multitude of live classes, thousands of on-demand classes, and scenic rides through the countryside that look absolutely gorgeous. You can customize your workouts using filters that provide a wide selection of rides that vary by length, intensity, style, music playlist, and even instructor. (Many Peloton instructors have become superstars in the cycling community. One of those instructors—Jenn Sherman—is perhaps the best known, not least because of the accolades she has received from radio personality Howard Stern. Robin Arzon, Peloton's VP of programming, is also immensely popular.)

Make no mistake about it, Peloton's instructors are the real deal. They are more than competent and engaging—which in my opinion ought to be the bare minimum. But these folks go above and beyond. For the sake of variety—and meeting the needs of all fitness levels—they each take a slightly different approach to their workouts. This really keeps riders coming back for more. And as you'll immediately find if/when you start using a Peloton, many instructors bring in their own DJs, which makes the class even more enjoyable and personalized!

The available Peloton classes range from beginner to advance beginner, low impact, interval, and climbing (which can be challenging and actually requires standing on the pedals). The versatility is really remarkable. Whether you're a beginner just looking to get back in shape or an experienced cyclist looking to really go hard and challenge yourself, there's going to be a class level that is right for you.

But what about accommodating your busy schedule? Some days you have more time than others. Well, Peloton's got you covered here, too.

In addition to intensity, the workouts can also be customized by time. The time ranges go from five minutes all the way up to two hours, but the majority of classes last between thirty and forty-five minutes.

Okay, I hear you saying, "It sounds like Peloton's got me covered when it comes to cycling and spinning exercises of all intensity levels. But what if I want something closer to a full-body workout? For what Peloton costs, I could be well on my way to affording a piece of home gym equipment that offers other exercises."

As you can probably guess, the pros at Peloton have thought of this, as well.

If you're looking for, say, an upper-body workout in addition to the cardio you're going to get on the bike, one-, two-, and three-pound dumbbells are available to complement many of the workouts, and they conveniently fit in a rack behind the Peloton's saddle. (It's important to note here that lifting while riding remains controversial within the spinning community; some feel that its more likely for riders—

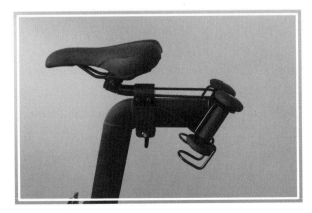

especially inexperienced ones—to injure themselves this way. As with all things I'm covering in this book, use common sense when deciding if it might be right for you and always consult with your doctor before beginning any new form of exercise program.)

At this point, a question that often comes up when I'm telling people about Peloton Bikes is "Can you pause a class if you need to use the restroom, or your child starts crying, or you drop your water bottle on the floor?" The answer is **NO**. At least not while taking a live or on-demand ride. Because of limitations in the technology, there is no way to stop them once they're started. (We can hope that one day Peloton will update the software to allow this—just as how live TV can be "paused" and then put on delay—yet for now, you can always rejoin the class, or start over from the beginning, after attending to whatever emergency arises.)

Yet another question I usually get from friends is about the safety and security of the investment. Sure, a Peloton Bike looks cool, works great, and has excellent HD content . . . but will it be around for a while? Moreover, if something were to somehow go wrong with my bike, would I be left out in the wilderness?

Here, Peloton has you covered. The included limited warranty that comes with all bikes covers the mechanics, tablet, and parts and service for all issues related to normal wear and tear occurring in the first year you own the bike. The bike's frame has a warranty of five years. If you're still concerned about the safety of your investment—maybe you live in a house with mischief-age children who might attack the bike—extended warranties are also available. (When it comes to making these extra warranties affordable, be on the lookout for referral codes that Peloton periodically offers. They can take up to one hundred dollars off of your costs.)

In addition, if you're fortunate enough to work at a company with a health insurance or wellness program that covers exercise programs, you may be able to get a reimbursement for the annual costs of using a Peloton Bike, just as you would for health clubs. Corporate policies about what employee wellness programs will cover are always shifting, but they seem to be moving in the direction of covering (at least partially) lively activities that will help keep workers healthy and fit. If you're not sure about your own workplace, my advice is to check with your company policy or Human Resources representative. And if they *don't* cover Peloton yet, let them know it's a benefit you desire. If enough employees express interest, management can often make adjustments accordingly.

While the custom, HD content is probably the "bread and butter" of how Peloton has transformed the home cycling experience, it's important to understand that the live (and prerecorded) classes aren't the only ways that Peloton harnesses technology to give you the best possible cycling experience.

While on the bike, you will be able to measure all sorts of health and fitness metrics, including ride time elapsed, ride time remaining, resistance, speed, cadence, distance covered, total output, calories burned, and your heart rate (if you wear a

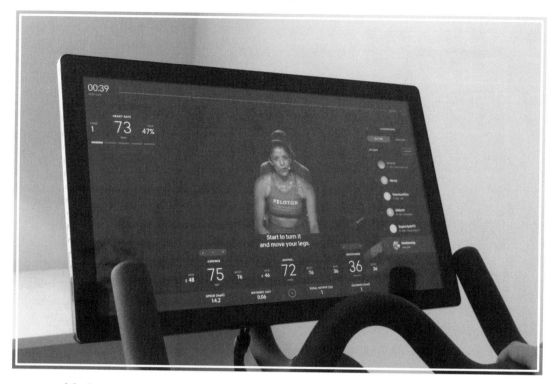

compatible heart monitor). These metrics aren't important to some users—who just want to enjoy a ride and not think about these specifics—and you're never compelled to unduly focus on them. But if you decide that you need them, Peloton makes getting your live metrics readout easy and intuitive.

In addition, a Leaderboard—located directly to the right of the HD screen—allows you to compare yourself to other people who are doing the same ride, in real-time, while you are in the saddle (or, if you like, against those riders who have taken that ride in the past). Some people thrive on this sort of friendly competition. Other riders dislike it. That's why Peloton keeps it completely optional and customizable.

And just like everything seems to these days, Peloton has an app. But while many products appear to have created an app out of peer pressure, or because they "feel they need to," Peloton has thoughtfully and carefully designed their app to truly complement the riding experience and bring enhancements that go above and beyond. On Peloton's app you'll find many of the same classes you can take while on the bike, but also thousands of additional classes in other categories related to fitness and wellness. You'll find sections for meditation and yoga, to enhance jogging or walking, and everything in between.

(Many of the people you pass on the street doing outdoor activities like running or cycling may be running the Peloton app through their earbuds.) Now, I

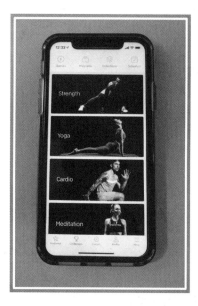

wouldn't invest in a Peloton exclusively for the app experience—the bike is still the star of the show—but if you're already interested in the bike, I think you'll find Peloton's app offerings to be a genuine value-add that helps create an excellent synergy with the other wellness activities you may choose to do.

So now that we've reviewed the good side of the technology, let me also address the main concern that Peloton buyers usually have—and that I certainly had, at least in the back of my mind—when it comes to technology. Namely, that it changes. Earlier I mentioned how VCRs led to a groundbreaking boom in home aerobics in the 1980s. But how many people still use their aerobics videocassettes today? How many people still have VCRs?

If you're thinking along these lines, you're not alone. But I hope I can convince you that there's excellent evidence that 1) Peloton is not going anywhere soon, 2) the technology Peloton uses now is cutting edge and is going to have a long and lasting impact in its space, and 3) that if and when home exercise technology does evolve once more, the odds are that Peloton will be one of the companies leading the way.

I'm no mathematician, but when I look at the comparatively high price of the bike ($2,200 and change) coupled with the monthly subscription costs (and the few, optional one-time costs for accessories), and I compare that with the annual fees of my health club—which might include the occasional hiring of a personal trainer, the price of spin classes in a studio, and how many people in my household would use it—I come to the conclusion that Peloton is worth the money. Moreover, Peloton's engineers are always updating their technology. The library of HD rides is always expanding. The number of accessories available for the bike is always increasing. The number of enhancements available on the app grows almost daily. When was the last time that your health club upgraded its equipment or facilities? And was that upgrade free, or did it involve an increase in membership dues?

Of course, the hesitation for some when it comes to pulling the trigger on a Peloton is the simple fact that companies can go out of business. (For those of you old enough to understand the reference, you may be saying: "Sure, VCRs were a hit . . . but how do I know I'm buying a VHS and not a Betamax?" Or: "Is this going to be the Blu-ray that becomes the dominant technology for a generation, or the HD-DVD that fizzles out in a few months?") I certainly don't blame people for wondering if there's a chance that Peloton maybe won't survive. If that happened, then yeah, the bike would be rendered pretty much useless (since there would be no more access to the subscription service, where all of the content is located). But I also think that after looking at the evidence, it would be downright silly to conclude that Peloton is going anywhere soon. A behemoth with a multibillion-dollar valuation, Peloton is poised to become a dominant force not just in spinning, but in fitness, period, in the coming years. It is expanding into new untapped markets, and its profile in our culture is only increasing. It has no serious competitors as a brand, and it utterly dominates its sphere of influence. There is no sense that the technology it uses could become redundant anytime soon.

If you still have questions related to Peloton as a sensible, long-term investment, I encourage you to make this book the start of your research, as opposed to the end of it. The assertions I've made here are backed up by virtually all fitness industry experts.

And if you're *still* nervous? Well, a Peloton is a big investment . . . but all I can say is that sometimes in life you have to take a chance.

For me, personally, when I think of the importance of my health, and the overall convenience that working out on a Peloton has afforded me—to say nothing of the psychological benefit I've enjoyed and the positivity that's come from knowing I'm investing in my own wellness—I just don't think I could put a price on it.

It's remarkable how seamlessly the Peloton has become a fixture in my life.

When I first wake up in the morning, I no longer look out the window or check my weather app to see if I need a coat. Nope. Instead, I go into the other room and work out on my Peloton. I honestly can't remember ever being this motivated to work out after the initial novelty of a device has worn off. For me, this adds a nice sort of "bookend" to the experience. Peloton the brand is in it for the long haul, and so am I. By keeping me engaged with high-end technology, an immersive experience, and classes that are custom and unique, Peloton has transcended what is typically called "workout equipment" and reached a whole other plane.

People with kids swear by Peloton because they don't have to spend needless time getting to and from the gym—and managing childcare in the process. For working people, Peloton makes it so easy to fit a workout into an already-busy day. But I think the biggest attraction has to be the way it removes the boredom and monotonous repetition that can be such a deterrent to exercise. Instead, it makes your daily, much-needed workout something that is new, different, and fresh every time. I think it's not an exaggeration to say that working out on a Peloton Bike can be a truly life-changing event.

Of course, I was not always a true believer. And I think there may be no more useful tale to tell here than the story of my own conversion . . .

* * *

A few weeks after leaving the Peloton store, my wife and I awaited the delivery of our new bike. Speaking frankly, we were excited—sure—but we were also praying that this new acquisition would not become an overpriced clothes rack one day.

My wife and I had reason to be worried. For years, we had had memberships at various gyms. Sometimes we took classes, or tried other enhancements to our workouts, but most of the time our memberships went unused. I don't know how much money we spent on time we simply never used at the gym, but it's certainly significant.

For me, I used to dread pulling myself out of bed and going to the gym on a cold, rainy morning. (Consequently, most of the time going to the gym "lost," and I'd roll over and go back to sleep.) And it wasn't just getting there. If I did make it to the gym, then it was boring with a capital *B*. It was not something I looked forward to. (I liked "having done it" but not actually doing it.) Working out was an intimidating, irritating, joyless experience.

The first clue that this time was going to be different was not just wishful thinking; it was when we got to know the people.

My wife and I have found that the employees who work for Peloton are very nice and exceedingly helpful. This was true in the showroom—sure—but find me a salesperson who isn't nice and helpful, and I'll show you somebody who's going to find a new line of work pretty soon. With Peloton, it's been consistent across everyone we've spoken with, listened to, or taken a class from.

As an example, the two people who delivered the bike to our home were knowledgeable and professional. They spent time making sure the bike was operating properly and gave us some tips on operating the bike before leaving. Just take a moment to consider how this customer service experience stacks up against what the American consumer has been conditioned to expect/tolerate. Even the most major, expensive purchases are frequently delivered to us by people unaffiliated with the company we're making the purchase from, and who don't know and/or don't care about the product itself.

But as good as our delivery and setup experience was, just days later when the first bill came due, I thought to myself: "This is a sizable chunk of change. If we'd been disappointed in the product—or if we'd had a lousy delivery and customer service experience—I'd be really upset at having spent all this money!"

I say this not to harp on the price of the machine, but instead to make this point: *If* you are going to make this type of investment—and, as I hope is clear, I think it is a very wise investment—then doesn't it make sense to demand the kind of product and service you get with Peloton? Doesn't it make sense to get everything you deserve out of the experience?

So now the bike was in our house. With all the ensuing excitement that came with receiving the delivery—not to mention the desire to start cycling right away—I confess that I might not have been paying the closest attention to all the details I was hearing during the setup. I expect I won't be the only one to experience this; it's a lot of information to take in all at once.

We live in exciting times when new technologies are being applied to consumer goods and services, and it seems as if our lives were constantly thereby improving. But at the same time, the speed of these advances can seem overwhelming at times. If you've purchased or leased a new automobile in the last five years—and it came "fully loaded"—then you know exactly what I am talking about. You can get in and start driving without a problem most of the time—sure—but how many hidden features are you unaware of? How many features are you *aware* that you're probably unaware of? To give a real example, when we got our last car, we drove around for literally *a couple of years* staring at the dashboard odometer until our son showed us how to initiate the car's head-on display. And on how many winter mornings did I handle a cold steering wheel before I finally discovered how to turn on the heated steering wheel function? (The answer is, more than I'd care to admit!) It's the same thing when it comes to new smartphones: we generally know how to make calls and text all right, but how many features do we discover gradually, over time, through trial and error?

Bear with me; all this is connected to my failure to listen closely as the Peloton's functions and nuances were explained to me.

The Peloton Bike is a beautifully crafted exercise machine. There's no doubt about that. The tablet that sits atop the handlebars is a work of ingenuity. But it is also a very advanced piece of exercise technology. Like so many contemporary electronic devices today, so much can be done with it that there simply isn't time to explore it all during delivery (or even in the store).

The good news is that when something doesn't work—or you have any kind of issue with the Peloton Bike—there are things you can do to troubleshoot those problems . . . if you just know how. There are things that are likely to occur with the bike, and things that are rare. And there are most certainly things you can discover about the bike and think to yourself (in a forehead-smacking sort of way): "If only I'd known that sooner!"

That is the reason I wanted to write this guide. I want you to learn what you'll need to know, and what you'll *want* to know. I want you to have a sense of what you ought to learn right away, and what you can bother with later. And I want you *never* to feel as though you were the only one experiencing certain issues when you're getting used to your Peloton Bike.

You could spend hours on the phone with Peloton support, surfing the web, watching YouTube tutorials (with long, ponderous introductions)—hey, at least you can use the Table of Contents to skip this one after reading it once!—or asking your friends what they would do in your situation. You *could*. But my goal is to make sure you won't have to. I want to help you quickly and effectively get the most out of your bike from the moment it enters your home. Though the Peloton Bike itself represents new, advanced technology, its tips and tricks can be well understood through one of the oldest technologies—the slim volume you hold in your hand.

The remainder of this book consists of PELO TIPS, which are based on topics that commonly come up—and issues you may experience—right after you get your bike home.

Within each tip, there are often many hacks, tricks, and subset pieces of advice all presented with a single goal in mind: *you* getting the *most* out of your Peloton Bike so you can easily and quickly begin reaching your desired fitness objective (and, just as important, so you can get straight to the *fun* parts of owning a Peloton).

It's one thing for me to talk about these tips, but quite another to show them to you. So without further ado, let's get underway!

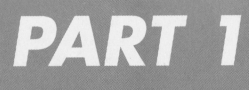

PART 1

GETTING THINGS SET UP

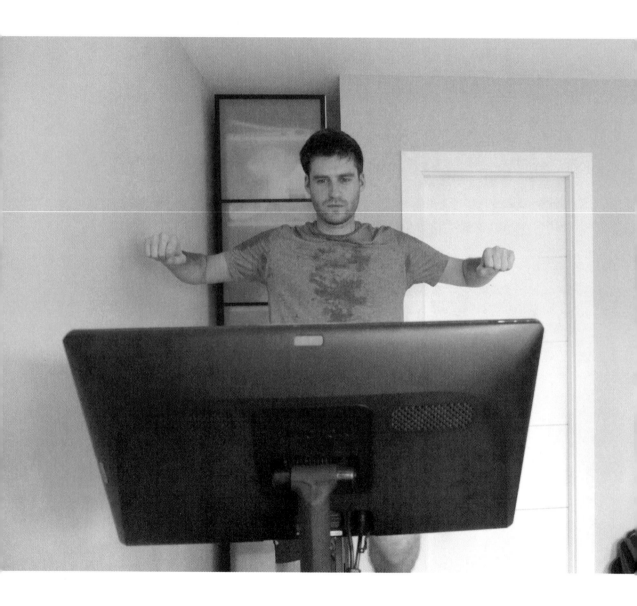

PELO TIP 1: PLACEMENT

One of the first things you will notice when you receive your bike (or when you look one over in the store) is that the Peloton Bike takes up relatively little space compared to other exercise machines. If you have only seen Peloton's television commercials, you may think that you'll need a large room (in a mansion with sweeping views of the ocean or mountains) in order to operate your bike comfortably. Nothing could be further from the truth!

I understand why Peloton's ad agency has chosen to block their shots this way—and to position the bikes in locales that are likely to add a little glamour to the brand—but a mansion room looking out on a mountaintop vista is optional.

At only four feet long and two feet wide, you can easily situate a Peloton Bike in the smallest of small apartments. And there's nothing wrong with positioning facing a wall. In fact, that actually might be the *best* place! You see, most of the time, your attention will be on an instructor (or scenic ride) being displayed on the twenty-two-inch tablet in front of you. Views that compete with the Peloton screen might actually be counterproductive (especially if you're an easily distracted person, like me).

If you do have a little extra space, it's optimal when positioning your Peloton to try to keep a clearance of at least two feet on either side of the bike. This is not only so you can get on and off the machine (and clip in and out of the pedals) more easily, but also so you won't knock anything over when extending your arms. As I noted earlier, Peloton workouts can often incorporate arm weights and/or stretching exercises. You'll want to be able to do these without worrying about hitting a wall!

Another question you will want to ask when it comes to positioning your Peloton Bike is "How good is the Wi-Fi?" This was something my wife and I had to adjust when we purchased our bike. Our initial placement location turned out to be fine for streaming classes, but we noticed there were connectivity problems when it came to screen-casting off-bike exercises on a television in another room. (More on troubleshooting this issue later.) But suffice to say, if you can position the Peloton close to your router, without any walls separating the two, it will probably optimize your overall experience.

PELO TIP 2: SURFACE

As something of a subset of the question "Where in my house should I put my bike?" I encourage you also to think about the physical *surface* you are going to be placing the bike on.

Many of us have homes with floor surfaces that vary. However, it is generally not a good idea to split your Peloton between types of flooring. For example, placing the front of the bike on a hardwood floor and the back on carpet or rug can result in the bike rocking and a funny, unstable feeling when you're riding. You'll want to avoid this, especially when you build your way up to the more challenging rides that involve lifting your body up off the saddle. It's okay to place the bike entirely on carpet, but it may take a short while for it to "settle in"—depending on the carpet's plushness. And make sure you're okay with deep indentations forming in the carpet/rug underneath your Peloton Bike, because, brother, it's going to happen. (Some people put a piece of plywood down beneath the carpet for this reason.) Most Peloton enthusiasts will tell you that solid, level floor is ideal, and many feel that hardwood floors are optimal. If you go this route, it is a good idea to use a high-density mat beneath the bike, so that you don't damage the bike or the floor. It doesn't necessarily have to be the high(er)-priced Peloton mat that the company offers for this purpose, but it should definitely be durable, textured, and slip-resistant (to prevent the bike from moving around). A mat also serves the helpful function of catching sweat for easy cleanup after a workout (and—believe me—you are going to sweat!), and it can also protect your floors from scratches if you wear clip-on cleats.

By taking a moment to find the optimal floor surface for your Peloton Bike, you'll help ensure that you get a comfortable ride and that you, your bike, and your flooring stay as safe and protected as possible.

PELO TIP 3: HOLD YOUR DELIVERY GUYS HOSTAGE. SERIOUSLY.

Most books about optimizing exercise equipment would not ask you to hold anybody hostage—even figuratively—but this is *not* most books.

The people who deliver your Peloton are going to be one of your biggest assets when it comes to getting the most out of your bike. They are also, paradoxically, going to be unlikely to want to stick around to answer questions and troubleshoot. This isn't personal. They're just busy. However, because of the knowledge they can provide, it's going to be *on you* to optimize your time with them.

Just like the sales personnel you'll encounter in the store at the mall, Peloton's delivery people are going to be extremely well trained, exceedingly polite, and very knowledgeable. That's the good news. The bad news is they are also very, very busy.

When the delivery people arrive at your residence, their goal is going to be to set up your new bike as quickly as possible, check to make sure everything is in working order, and give you just enough basics on the bike (such as adjusting the seat and handlebars and making sure your touch screen tablet is functioning correctly) to get you flying under your own power, so to speak. The moment that's done, they'll need to rush off to their next delivery in order to meet their quota for the day.

Now, it's possible that you'll be among those Peloton customers who are completely in tune with all the latest technology and who never have any mechanical issues with a piece of equipment. If that's the case, more power to you! But if you're the kind of person who sometimes needs a nudge in the right direction when it comes to technology, you'll want to make sure you maximize your time with the delivery people.

The first best practice for maximizing your time is to **know exactly where you want them to install the bike** and **have your home Wi-Fi username and password handy**. Hemming and hawing on either of these while the techs wait around is a very bad use of your time with them.

My next tip is to **pay close attention to what the people setting up your bike say to you!** It would not be unreasonable for you to consider recording them on your phone, or for you to take written notes regarding what they have to say.

Even assuming that you are a quick study—and already accustomed to using things like Wi-Fi and Bluetooth on your devices—it is more than likely that in your excitement to get this beautiful piece of machinery set up so you can start riding, you might not be in the right mindset to pay close attention to the rapid-fire instructions that these delivery people are giving you (and largely doing by rote). It is also possible that shortly after they leave—even if you've been paying close attention—you'll have forgotten all the important things they said. Hey, it happens to the best of us! So take notes. Take a video. And really listen to what the bike techs are telling you.

If you do this, you will maximize the time available for questions, which is what you really want to do.

The game is to keep them at your house as long as possible. Would I tell you to be above stooping to reliable tricks to make them stick around? If that's what you think, then you're reading the wrong kind of Peloton book!

One way to make your bike tech linger (and answer questions) is to offer them a beverage—which they will certainly be grateful for. Offer to let them use the bathroom, or offer them a snack if it's handy. Think of them as a guest you're trying to get to linger for just a bit longer.

Another—and perhaps more controversial tactic in this connection—is to **offer a gratuity right out of the gate**. If it feels awkward to hand someone a a twenty-dollar bill the moment they put down the bike, there are ways to be more subtle about it. One way to signal that you will be tipping your Peloton delivery person is to put the money out in a conspicuous place. You want them thinking that if they answer all your questions and really take their time with you, it is going to be worth it to them. (I recognize that some might take umbrage at needing to tip these delivery people at all. If this bike was a major purchase for you—which it probably was—and you've already shelled out "a lot of money," then the last thing you want to do is spend more. But even if you're somebody who doesn't usually tip service people, I encourage you to make an exception here. It's hard for me to think of a tip that is better spent!)

By keeping the delivery person around longer, your brain will have more time to process everything—and it will seem like a lot—as they patiently explain the wonders of your new purchase. You'll have time to ask questions about the bike that may be unique to you, and which I can't anticipate in this book! I really encourage you to make the most of it.

PELO TIP 4: ADJUSTING SEAT AND HANDLEBARS

Getting the correct adjustment for your bike's seat and handlebars is absolutely key. These are the parts of the bike that will actually touch your body the most. If you're not comfortable with them, then the overall Peloton experience is probably going to be frustrating and lacking.

There are two settings on your seat that you can adjust: the height and the depth. If you want to adjust the height, find the lever located partway down the seat shaft, just over the pedals. Start making the adjustment by turning the lever to the left. Raise or lower the seat until it is aligned to your hip bone (when you're standing aside the bike). Then tighten the setting by moving the lever to the right.

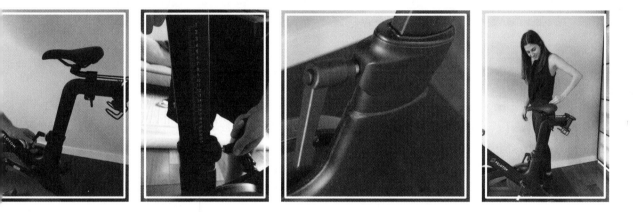

To adjust for depth, turn the lever that is directly located under the seat to the left. This will allow you to move the seat forward or backward. A good rule of thumb for making this setting is to bend your arm and place your elbow against the nose of the seat, while extending your fingers to make sure they touch the handlebar. Again, when you've got a setting you like, tighten the lever by turning it to the right.

To adjust the handlebar, loosen the lever at the very front of the bike. After you've done that, straddle the bike in front of the seat. Then hold your arms under the handlebar and lift it into a comfortable position—then tighten the lever. It is recommended that you start off your Peloton experience by raising the handlebar to the highest possible level. Then, through trial and error, you can adjust it again and again until you find the optimal comfortable height.

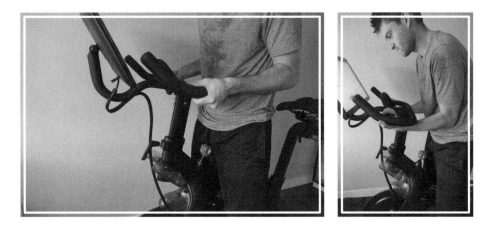

PELO TIP 5: THERE'S A LEVER IN THE WAY!

Part of riding a Peloton Bike is embracing the fact that levers can get in the way. By "in the way" I don't merely mean in an ugly position in terms of cosmetics of the bike. I mean in the way of a safe and fun ride. Obviously, having something that interrupts the comfort and intended orientation of your bike can be a barrier to the kind of Peloton experience you're looking for. The good news is that Peloton's engineers have done a fine job of making almost every part of the bike adjustable. So if a lever is sticking out at a weird angle, simply pull the lever out and turn it down to the 6 o'clock position. This should solve your problems. Moreover, if a lever looks wrong, take the time to do this fix. You'll be glad you did, and you'll avoid risking frustration and injury.

PELO TIP 6: MULTIPLE RIDERS

Is there a chance that you're going to be in one of the thousands of households that purchases a Peloton "because we'll both use it" or even "for the whole family"? There's no question that sharing a Peloton can absolutely help you to defray/reconcile the cost of the bike in dollars. And the good news is that Peloton has made it easy to adjust the bike when more than one person will be using it.

Unless you're sharing an apartment with your identical twin, the people in your household using the Peloton are going to have to use the levers to adjust the seat and handlebars to fit their bodies each time they use it. A simple best practice (at first) is to write down your individual seat height and depth and the handlebar height so you don't have to figure it out each time. This will save time when you are ready to jump on and start riding. (It can also be a nice thing to do to adjust the bike back to the settings of the other person who uses the bike when you're done!) After a short while, you'll have your settings memorized, and adjusting the bike to your personal specifications will come quickly and easily.

PELO TIP 7: SENSITIVE BUTTS . . . AND BITS

In my experience, the world of Peloton riders is largely divided into two camps. There are those who feel that the default Peloton seat is the most comfortable they have ever experienced on a bicycle . . . and there are those for whom it is literally a "sore subject."

Those in the first camp swear up and down that after six or seven rides, you won't feel anything. Your body will adjust and the seat will feel natural. Certainly, they insist, you won't have any pain in the butt or private parts.

But I am in the second camp. To me, the Peloton's default seat—if not exactly painful to sit upon—is definitely not the most comfortable. For those of us in this camp, I strongly recommend investing in padded shorts as a solution. Good padded shorts are made of spandex, lycra nylon, and polyester. They are lightweight and sweat absorbent, and the soft fiber offers unrestricted movement on the bike. Contemporary padded shorts are reinforced

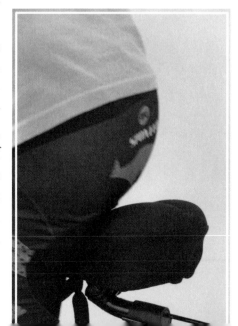

with 3D high-density foam mixed with silicone gel. For not too much money, you can get a pair of these bad boys and see that the pain to your backside and privates is drastically reduced (if not eliminated completely).

If you really want to go crazy—or you're just really passionate about comfort—you can also get a bike gel seat cover that will stick to your saddle. That extra cushion makes riding easier and may help you reach your goals without worrying about posterior pain.

If the Peloton experience feels A-OK to you with none of these enhancements, then all the better for you. But if you experience slight (or significant) discomfort when riding, I encourage you to go for one of these easy fixes!

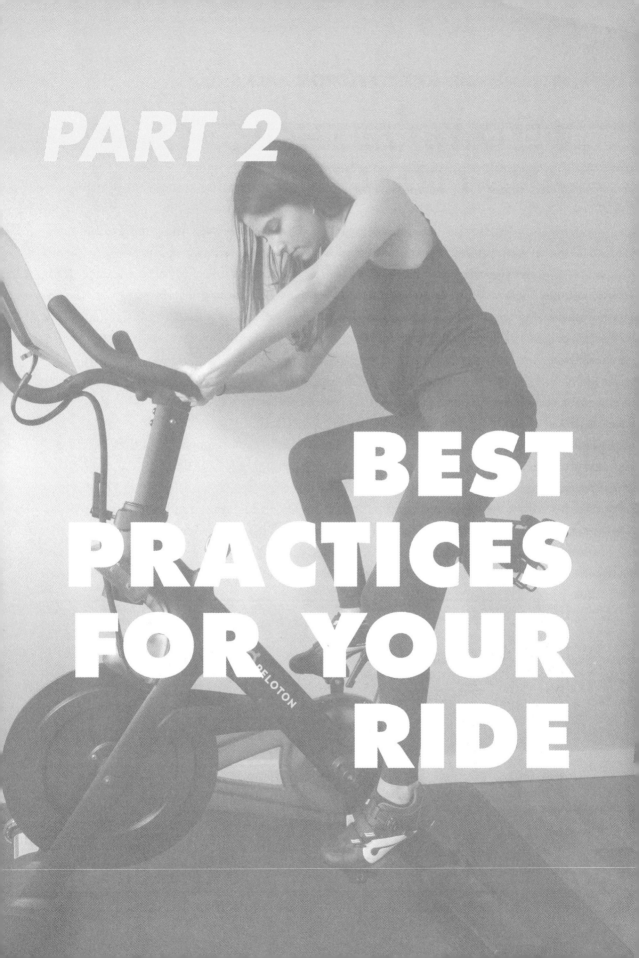

PART 2

BEST PRACTICES FOR YOUR RIDE

PELO TIP 8: SHOES, CLEATS, AND PEDALS

In Season ten, episode one, of HBO's hit comedy show *Curb Your Enthusiasm*, Larry David is on his Peloton Bike when his doorbell rings. To those of us who are already Peloton obsessives, we notice right away that Larry is not clipped in. He gets off the bike easily in this scene, because he is wearing regular exercise shoes.

This might seem like a small, insignificant detail to notice, but it's actually connected to the first big decision you'll make as a Peloton owner: your personal preference for footwear during your rides.

If you're not yet aware, you'll be happy to know that the pedals on a Peloton can be customized: there are those that accommodate the Peloton branded cleats, other spin class shoes, or sneakers.

Typically, a new bike comes equipped with stock pedals compatible with Look Delta Cleats. These cleats are made of extra-strong, heavy-duty engineering thermoplastic. They fit well with the pedal and have a three-hole arrangement that allows for enhanced stability. The shoe itself is quite comfortable. In addition to two Velcro straps, it comes with a ratchet strap to make it snug and also has a release button that is easy to use. When you put the notched strap through the plastic section, you can then tighten by lifting the lever on it, once for each notch. When you want to loosen

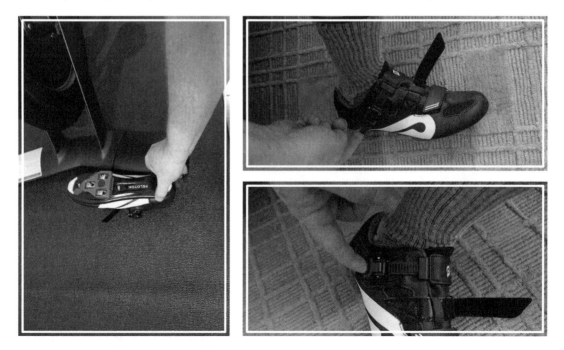

it, push the smaller lever on the release button and pull the notched strap away from the plastic section. The system is easy and intuitive.

But maybe using the default cleats is not your speed. In that case, another option is to attach toe cages to the pedal. This will allow you to wear your own sneakers (or whatever you like) as you ride your Peloton.

People who have ridden other exercise bikes might already have Shimano Pedaling Dynamic (SPD) cleats. These do not work with the stock Peloton pedals. But, interestingly, commercial Peloton Bikes in hotels and many gyms offer bikes with the SPD pedals on one side of the gym, and those with sneaker cages on the other side.

My wife and I use the Peloton shoes, and although there was a learning curve when it comes to getting in and out, we have come to love them. Our son, on the other hand, uses his sneakers without a toe cage. Though this means his feet slip from time to time, he still enjoys his workouts.

Finally, I ought to note that there seems to be a widely acknowledged psychological benefit—or, at least, a "psychological effect"—to being clipped in. It makes people feel "in the zone" for their workout, and is a healthy deterrent to outside influences. There is something to be said for committing to a ride and not stopping your ride to answer the phone or go to the door like Larry David. This is your time to exercise, and nothing should distract you from your workout goals.

PELO TIP 9: CLIPPING IN AND CLIPPING OUT

As you can probably guess by this point in the book, on the day our new bike arrived, my wife and I were very eager to give it a spin. She decided to go first while I was at work.

Putting on her new Peloton shoes, she somehow managed to click in after a few tries, despite struggling with the pedal. She then enjoyed a twenty-minute beginners class. But when that class ended, my wife's first-day troubles began.

No matter how much she tried, she couldn't clip out. She was literally trapped on the bike! Pulling her phone off the water bottle tray, she tried calling me at the office, but I was in a meeting and the call went to voicemail.

When I got home that night, what greeted me was like a scene out of a horror film or a crime novel. Her shoes were on the pedals . . . but the rest of her was nowhere to be found. It was *The Case of the Disappearing Peloton Wife!* (Luckily, my fears were unfounded. My wife had just stepped out of her shoes.)

It's a silly story, but it makes an important point. What we learned from this experience is that, generally speaking, clicking in is relatively easy. When sitting on your bike, you use your foot to rotate one pedal toward the floor until you get to the six-o'clock position. Below the handlebar is a large orange knob. If you then push down on the knob, the pedals will lock. (The same thing happens if you turn the knob all the way to the right.) Locking pedals makes it easier to clip in or out.

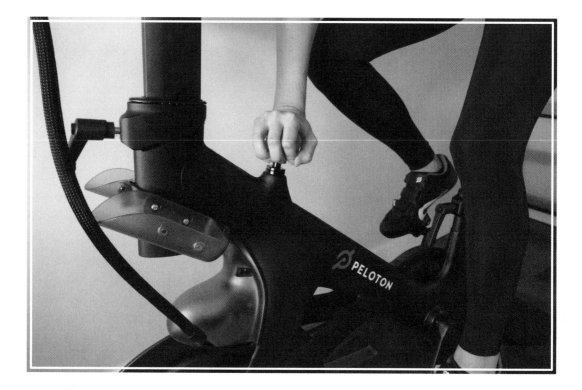

When you're looking to clip in effectively, you'll want to center the Delta cleat (on the bottom of your shoe) as best as you can below the toes, directly over the Delta-shaped cutout on the pedal. (Note the white "Peloton" word is stamped on the heel of the pedal.) Make sure your foot is aligned straight with the bike, then move your toes forward and push down on your heel until it snaps in place. Make sure you hear a click.

Repeat with your other cleat and pedal. If you have ever skied, it is a similar feeling to putting your boot in the binding.

But that's just clipping in . . . the thing my wife **didn't** have a problem with.

When your workout is over, and you are ready to disembark the bike, begin by once again rotating the pedal toward the floor to the six-o'clock position and locking the orange knob. Then, keeping your toes forward, push down on your heel and move your heel and ankle out to the side. Don't be afraid to apply pressure when you make this motion.

This motion isn't complicated, per se, but after a workout it can be easier said than done.

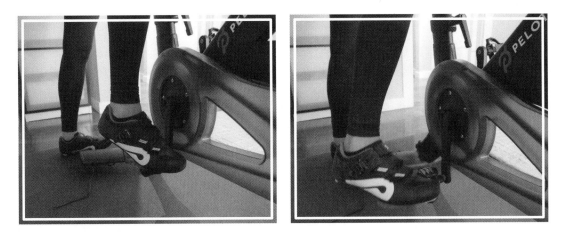

Sometimes you're going to be tired from the ride, and your leg and foot are going to be shaky. Or something may have happened that has made you anxious to get off the bike quickly. Ironically, both of these make it harder to do the very thing you intend to do—which is to clip out and get off the bike.

When this happens, don't panic. Remain calm. Take a deep breath and try to steady your leg. (I think you'll be surprised how much forcing yourself to slow down helps.) Then focus on your toes and heel, and your foot will come out more easily.

Moving to a slightly less serious aspect, I should note that there is no general agreement regarding which foot one should clip out first. I encourage you to go with what's most natural for you. Personally, I am a righty. My bike is situated close to a wall on the right side. I feel comfortable clipping out on that side first. Then, when I'm finished with the right foot, I swing that leg over the saddle, which makes it super easy for the left foot to come out.

Everyone masters clipping in and out at different rates, so don't worry if it takes a little time for you to perfect. Some Peloton riders recommend looking at the bottom of the pedal, where there is a tension screw. You can turn this screw a little to loosen it to get your foot out. However, Peloton officially cautions people against clipping out this way, because if you loosen the screw too much, it's possible to break the pedal. However, at least anecdotally, it seems that for some new riders, it remains the best way to disengage from the bike. So if you feel that you must use this tactic, I recommend that you make very small, incremental changes to the tension screw. Go cautiously and gingerly to avoid doing any permanent damage to your bike.

In conclusion, don't let clipping in and out be more intimidating than it needs to be. Trust me when I say: after a few times clipping in and out, it will be as easy as saying your ABCs!

PELO TIP 10: POSITIONING AND ERGONOMICS

Now let's move away from accessories and get to something even more fundamental: positioning and configuring your bike itself.

When it comes to getting on and off your Peloton Bike, the old adage of "no pain/no gain" does not apply here. I can't stress this enough: to get the most out of your Peloton Bike, you'll need to be comfortable. You don't burn any more calories or increase your heart rate to a greater degree simply because you are in ergonomic discomfort. To the contrary, having your bike configured in a way that causes you unnecessary pain is antithetical to your workout goals, because it will make you less likely to push yourself (or even to ride the bike at all). That's why it's vital to take the time to position and orient your bike to make sure it's calibrated for your body.

It's easy to see if your bike is configured correctly. After clicking into your bike, with your hands lightly on the handlebar, bring your right pedal to the six-o'clock position. Your knee should have a slight bend. If you don't have a bend, lower the seat. Conversely, if you have too much of a bend in your knee—and it feels like an awkward overextension—simply raise the seat.

Now try moving your pedal to the three-o'clock position. Your knee should be above the area between your toes and the arch of your foot. If it isn't, you should adjust the seat either forward or back until you feel that your knee is correctly aligned.

Your own comfort should be paramount when configuring your bike. If something looks right but feels wrong, then it's wrong! When you pedal, it should feel comfortable. Your butt should be back in the saddle and you should feel "strapped in," figuratively speaking. Your hips should not be rocking back and forth, and you should not be straining to reach the bottom of each pedal stroke. (Straining and reaching are a problem because you could bruise your groin or develop lower back pain by repeating these strained motions. To correct a position that makes you feel like you are reaching and strained, try lowering the seat incrementally until you feel you've achieved the right comfort level. Again, if it feels right, then there's a 99 percent chance it is right.)

When you start using your Peloton, it may be worth your time to take notes regarding which positions and settings work for you. If you're "on the fence" about whether a particular setting is optimal or not, write notes about how you feel after a ride. Compare these notes with others you make after trying rides in different settings. These sorts of small "trial-and-error" approaches can end up providing the info you need to find the optimal settings for your Peloton.

PELO TIP 11: RIDING POSTURE

The correct posture for riding an exercise bike is by no means intuitive, especially for first-time riders., It's important to do your best to go into a Peloton ride with the physical posture that most likely will prevent injury and keep you riding for longer.

The biggest area in which riders make a mistake regarding their posture involves the bike's handlebars. The handlebars are only there to help you balance, but that's it. They aren't meant to be load bearing. When you're riding your Peloton, resist the urge to hunch over and have the handlebars bear the entire weight of your upper body. The thing that should be keeping you upright isn't the handlebars; it's you.

In addition to leaning on them excessively, another issue with the handlebars can be grip. Certainly, there are exciting parts of certain Peloton workouts where you're going to want to grip the handlebars more enthusiastically. This is normal and appropriate. However, if you grip the handlebars too tightly during the entire ride, it can result in unnecessary tension in your back and shoulders. Gripping tightly to keep balanced probably means that the bike has not been set up correctly to fit your body type. If you are doing it right and have the correct handlebar height, you should have only a slight bend in your elbows, and you shouldn't feel the need to constantly grip hard.

There is also the question of where to grip the handlebar. The answer: on the widest parts.

During your initial Peloton classes, your instructor will often remind you of proper positioning of your hands on the handlebar. Later on, when you've moved up to slightly more advanced classes, you may be instructed to move the orange resistance knob to the right, which will simulate the feeling of climbing a hill. Your instructor might suggest that you raise yourself out of the seat to do this. Your head should be held high, your shoulders back, and your hands lightly on the handlebars for balance. As you stand, your hips should be just over the pedals. It can take some time to get comfortable with standing up in the saddle, and you may need to build up stamina to do it well. That's okay. Don't feel frustrated; the instructors each have their own vocabulary and set of encouragements to help you master this position. Listen to them and follow their advice, and in no time you'll be riding (and standing up) with the best of them.

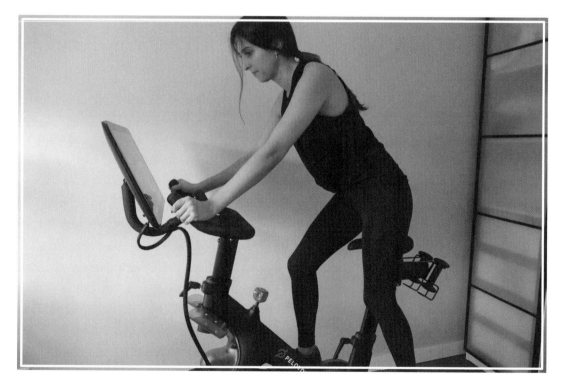

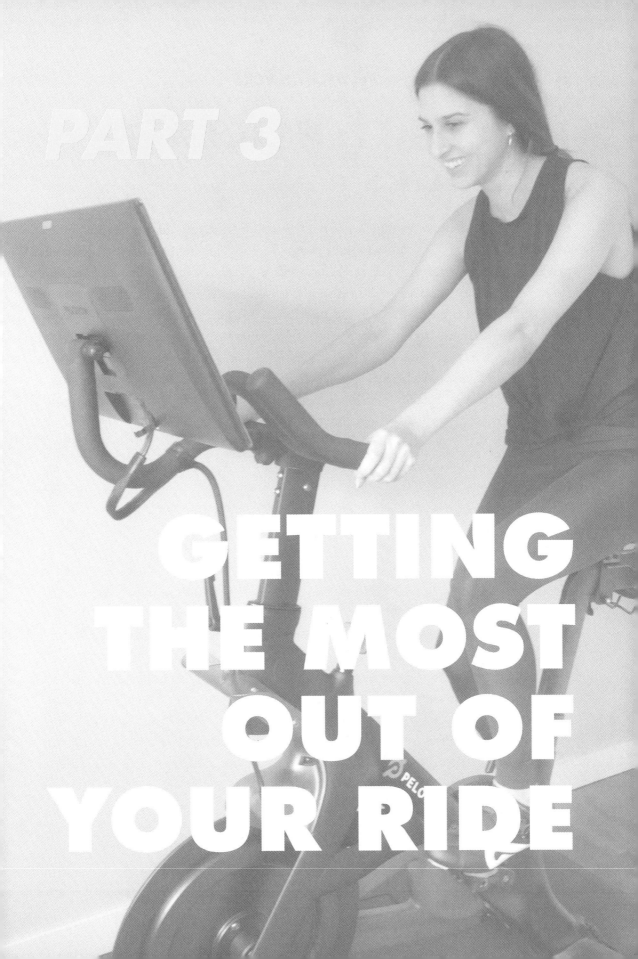

PART 3

GETTING THE MOST OUT OF YOUR RIDE

PELO TIP 12: HEART RATE MONITORS

Part of the fun of a Peloton Bike is tracking your progress, and taking full advantage of all the technology that the product offers. There are various metrics that you will probably want to observe as you set your workout goals. If you are like most Peloton riders, one of these metrics—either initially or eventually—will be heart rate.

I strongly recommend wearing a heart rate monitor in order to get the most out of your workout. There are many quality monitors on the market that are made precisely for activities such as riding an exercise bike. A lot of people swear by a monitor called the Scosche Rhythm. It wraps comfortably around your arm, and in addition to monitoring your beats per minute (BPM,) it displays your blood flow and how many calories you've burned. Other favorites are devices by Garmin, Wahoo, and Cat Eye. These are all quality brands that offer solid functionality. Whichever one you ultimately choose, just make sure to select a device with ANT+ technology; this allows several devices to communicate with one another and ensures that products from multiple brands can work together. For example, an ANT+ heart rate strap can send data to a bike, computer, watch, phone, or tablet— regardless of the manufacturer.

As you might imagine—given their popularity and ubiquity—Peloton offers its own monitors. My wife and I bought the Peloton Heart Rate Monitor as part of a package that also included shoes, mat, and headphones. If you're looking to hit the ground running with a monitor, this may be a quality option for your household, as well.

To wear the Peloton Heart Rate Monitor, you first snap the sensor pod into the chest strap. You can then adjust the strap to fit your lower chest. It should be snug but comfortable. When the heart rate monitor detects a heartbeat, the LEDs will flash red and blue. (The initial red flash indicates it detects the heartbeat, and it will stop flashing after thirty seconds. The flashing blue indicates it detects a heartbeat, and also that it is in Bluetooth pairing mode. The LED will continue flashing until the monitor connects to a Bluetooth device, even if you connect to the Peloton Bike via ANT+).

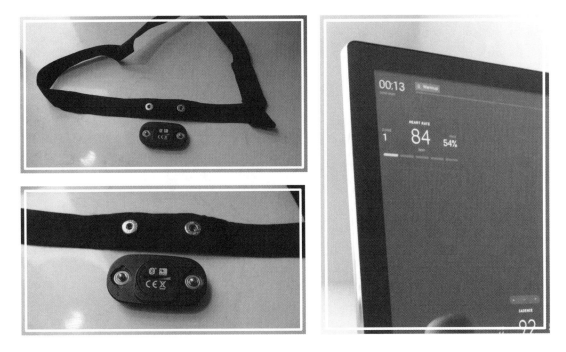

And if you see a flashing yellow light? Don't worry! It just means that the heart rate monitor's battery is low. You can replace it quickly and easily with a new CR2032 3-volt battery. The battery door is located on the underside of the sensor pod. Unscrew it by inserting a coin into the slot and rotating it counterclockwise. Once the door is loose, simply remove it. The battery is located just inside. Take out the old battery and wait thirty seconds. Then insert a new CR2032 3-volt battery with the flat side facing down. Replace the battery door and—with the coin in the slot—rotate clockwise until the door is flush with the underside of the pod.

You won't see the yellow light too frequently. The battery life for the Peloton Heart Rate Monitor is approximately six hundred hours.

You will notice that sometimes the red and blue lights on your monitor will flash even if you are not wearing the strap. This might happen just from touching the sensors on the strap, or because of the monitor's proximity to the bike. I recommend you unsnap the sensor pod from the chest strap when you are not riding. It is an easy enough thing to do so you will not waste time when you next go to exercise.

PELO TIP 13: WHAT TO DO WHEN THE HEART RATE MONITOR DISAPPEARS FROM YOUR SCREEN

Though the technology in your Peloton Bike is certainly leading-edge, it isn't perfect; there are still a few quirks to look out for. They aren't serious, just annoying. But learning to expect them, and handling them when they do pop up, is key to a quality Peloton experience. And of all the small technology quirks you may notice, the most common is simply that you'll get on the bike and be all clipped in and ready to go . . . but your heart rate isn't anywhere to be found on the screen. (Or else it will appear briefly and just as suddenly disappear.)

When this occurs, you might see a pop-up notice that your heart rate monitor has disconnected—but also, you might not. Don't be alarmed if this happens . . . it simply means it's time to troubleshoot.

The first—and most common—source of the problem is found within the Bluetooth connection to your bike. To explore this possibility, tap on the tablet screen once. Then, in the upper right-hand corner, tap on "Settings." Scroll down to the "Heart Rate Monitor" and make sure the Bluetooth setting is lit-up/on. If it is, and you still don't see your device listed on the screen, try turning it off for twenty seconds and then turning it on again. It should now indicate that the monitor is connected.

If the monitor is still not found, power off the tablet using the gray button on the backside of the tablet at the very top. Then, after waiting twenty seconds, boot it up once more. Many Peloton users have found that this simple restart method often gets the heart rate monitor function working again.

Finally, a less-frequent source of the issue can be the physical heart rate monitor itself. Sometimes you have to moisten the sensors that touch your chest in order to get the monitor working. If adjusting the tablet itself has not worked, try this technique and see if it gets the desired effect.

PELO TIP 14: HEART RATE ZONES

Learning about heart rate zones can be a key part of getting the most from your Peloton Bike experience. It's certainly a feature with which I wish I had acquainted myself sooner!

I had ridden for a couple of weeks before exploring it. While I thought I understood how my heart rate was connected to the rides I was doing, I kept seeing different "Zones" show up on the tablet screen, and I had no idea what that meant. But after doing some research on the Internet, I discovered that this Zones feature could offer a whole other dimension to my rides.

It turns out that Peloton offers a tool that allows you to take part in what they call "heart rate training." Peloton breaks down this training into five different zones, each of which corresponds to a specific level of effort. The percentages of each zone are based on your Maximum Heart Rate (MHR).

This is how Peloton describes it:

Zone 1
Warm Up
Up to 65% of MHR
This is an easy effort, like a warm-up or recovery.

Zone 2
Endurance
65-75% of MHR
This is an average effort, which is characterized as comfortable.

Zone 3
Power
75-85% of MHR
This is an above-average effort, which is characterized by heavy breathing.

Zone 4
Threshold
85-95%
This is a hard effort, characterized as very challenging.

Zone 5
Max Capacity
95%+ of MHR
As hard as you can manage, and it is characterized as a short burst to the finish line.

As you ride with your monitor on, your heart rate and current Zone will be displayed on the touch screen. But no sooner will you see this than you'll wonder—just as I did—how Peloton can possibly know this information for each individual rider. Every Peloton user's fitness level is different, after all. How does Peloton get a sense of the average rider's cardiovascular strength, versus someone who has, say, ridden in the Tour de France?

It turns out that there are several ways that Peloton comes by this information. If you filled out your profile when the installer was setting up your touch screen, you probably entered your birth date (unless you lied about your age). This is one metric from which Peloton will glean info about you. The bike also takes into account your fitness level as customized by your own adjustments to the rides. Whenever you feel that a ride is too easy or too difficult, you can adjust things by tapping the "Menu" on the bottom right-hand corner of your screen. Scroll down to "Max Heart Rate" and tap on it. This will lead to a screen that gives you two choices: you can keep it on default calculation, or you can enter your own custom MHR.

Peloton also offers heart rate training classes in the on-demand library, which you can easily search for. As I said in the introduction, this bike is full of nice surprises!

PELO TIP 15: HEART RATE MONITOR STRAP

There's nothing like a good ride on your Peloton to work up a lot of sweat. This is something for which you should be prepared.

When you take off your heart rate monitor, as noted above, you'll want to unsnap the monitor pod to preserve the battery. But what of the strap? To be frank, there's a good chance that your strap is going to be drenched with sweat. If you're like a lot of riders, you will be tempted to let it dry off on the bike handlebar. There's nothing wrong with that—per se—but the salt content in your perspiration will start to harden the strap and stain it over time. This means you'll have to replace your strap more frequently. A better idea is to rinse the strap under running water after a workout, and even clean the strap gently with mild soap (such as dish soap) every once in a while. (Do not soak, iron, or dry-clean it and avoid using moisturizing soaps because they can leave residue on the strap.) By keeping your strap clean and sweat-free, you'll have a nicer riding experience.

PELO TIP 16: TOWELS

While we are on the subject of sweating, let's talk about towels. I think it's a great idea to keep a small hand towel on the handlebar of your bike while you ride. If you're interested in investing in official equipment, there is a two-piece towel set (made of terrycloth) designed specifically for the Peloton handlebars, and a separate wiping towel to protect the bike from moisture. Personally, that seems to be a little excessive to me—and an area where I didn't feel each and every one of my riding accessories needed to be "on brand"—but to each his or her own. (I won't pass judgment on you if you decide to purchase a fancy Peloton sweat towel, if you don't pass judgment on me for getting the padded shorts AND the padded seat cover!)

PELO TIP 17: HYDRATE

We all know the importance of adequate hydration—and not just when exercising. When you're doing a ride on your Peloton, you're going to want to take small steps ahead of time to make it easy and intuitive to stay hydrated. It's a good idea to put a water bottle on the tray just below the handlebars for every ride. If you prefer, you can use a good sports energy drink to replace the electrolytes you will lose during your workout. At a minimum, you should take two or three gulps of water for every ten to fifteen minutes of your ride (and certainly keep drinking after you finish, as you feel you need to). Occasionally, during some rides, you will see a water bottle-shaped icon appear on your screen. This indicates that Peloton recommends this moment for taking some hydration.

It's true that riding a bicycle while taking a drink of water is not something that comes naturally to everybody. (In a perfect world, I might use a sippy cup, but even

I have my pride.) The best solution I have found is a leak-proof bottle that has a one-handed flip top that gives you quick and easy access so you don't have to miss a thing on your ride. When selecting a water bottle, go for ease of use. You want to be able to click the button with a finger and tip up the spout without any effort, and easily snap it closed when you are done.

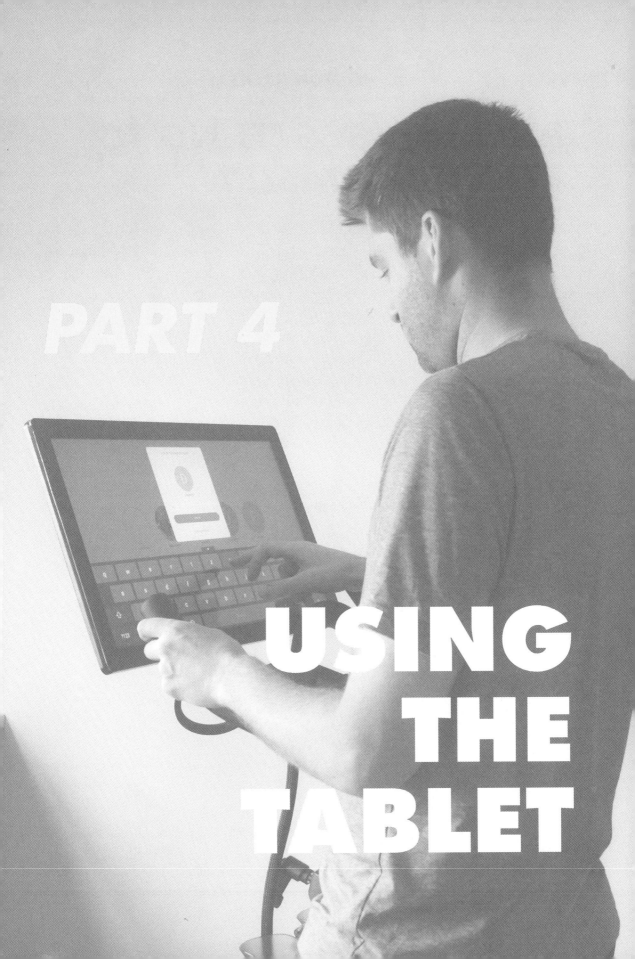

PART 4

USING THE TABLET

PELO TIP 18: GETTING TO KNOW THE TABLET

As I hope I've made clear by this juncture, the touch screen tablet on your bike is a pretty sophisticated piece of equipment. While you're enjoying riding your Peloton Bike, the tablet is collecting data and accessing and analyzing that information. By getting to know your tablet, you can make sure that you get the most out of this powerful tool and make it work for you.

For starters, let me say that you shouldn't be afraid to tap around on your tablet; it is pretty hard to mess it up. Explore it however you see fit.

Let me take you through my own experience with the tablet. My wife and I keep our bike in sleep mode. It's programmed to automatically go into that mode after five minutes of inactivity. When I tap twice on the tablet screen, the first thing I see is the "Choose Profile" page, containing icons for each user in our household. I tap once on my username and get to the home page. In the upper right I'll see a box notifying me of an upcoming live ride that I can join. Below that will be a number of recommended on-demand classes, challenges, and programs. There is certainly no shortage of choices.

Then, on the bar at the bottom of the screen, from left to right you'll see the following:

- Your personal page: this contains an overview of your personal stats, calendar, workout history, achievements, graphs highlighting your activities, and music you might have saved during rides.
- Your home page.
- Programs that group different classes by theme, instructor, music, fitness level, and mood.

When it comes to programs—especially if you're new to Peloton—I would advise starting with the "Welcome to Peloton Cycling" series. This is a collection of eighteen beginner classes, each running for about twenty minutes. These offer an excellent way to get comfortable with cycling on a Peloton and also introduce you to different instructors (whom you may like so much that you'll seek out their other classes).

On your tablet display, just to the right of programs, you will find classes. These

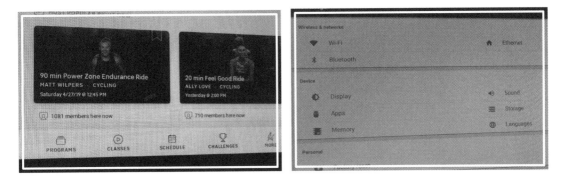

classes are intuitively organized by instructor, length, music genre, class type, subtitles, and weights.

Meanwhile, over on the schedule tab, you'll see that you can make appointments for upcoming live classes you'd like to attend. Peloton will even send you a reminder of upcoming classes at your email address.

The next tab you'll see contains active challenges that are coming up, if you are feeling especially goal-oriented.

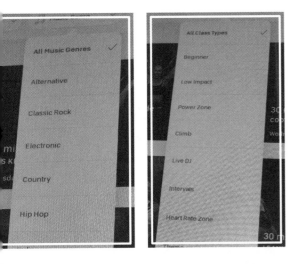

Whenever you tap the "More" tab, you are given two choices:

"Just Ride," which is the place to go to do your own thing and record your metrics.

The other choice will be "Scenic Rides," which gives you a choice to ride all over the world on country roads, city streets, off-road mountain bike simulation, or a combination thereof.

Personally, I love to vary my days. For example, one day I will take a live or

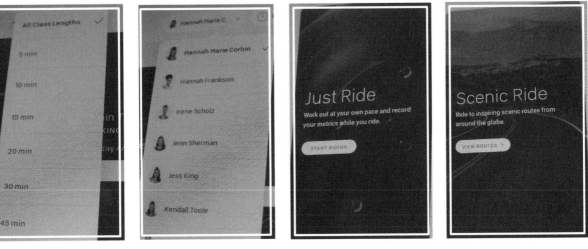

on-demand class with one of the instructors I like, and on the alternate days I will do a scenic ride. This way it never gets boring for me. I hope you'll find you have the same experience!

Your tablet's screen also functions in an interactive way. To the right you'll see a "Message Center" that has recommendations from fellow Peloton travelers.

The final tab—all the way to the right on the bottom of the tablet screen—is a menu that takes you to a master menu of functions that includes:

- Instructors
- Peloton Members
- Facebook Friends
- Profile Settings
- Device Settings
- Peloton 101
- Get Help
- About
- Log Out

Then, on the upper right of your screen you'll see the Wi-Fi strength indicator, a clock set to your local time, and settings. To make changes here, tap on settings, and a drop-down menu will allow you to change Wi-Fi settings, brightness, volume, cast screen, Bluetooth audio, heart rate monitor, and device settings.

I hope that the depth and breadth of functions is inspiring, not intimidating. I gave the example of a car earlier, and I think it applies here again. You don't need to know every function on the dashboard in order to drive the car, and you don't need to master every function available on your Peloton in order to have a great riding experience. I encourage you to do what my wife and I did: explore it at your own pace. Don't try to learn everything on the first day. Instead, accept that it will be a gradual and unique journey to getting the most out of your bike.

PELO TIP 19: THE LEADERBOARD

So, whether you are taking a class or going on a scenic ride, you're going to see all sorts of numbers when you ride your Peloton. At the bottom of your screen will be three numbers with which you will become very familiar over the course of owning your Peloton Bike:

- To the left, you'll see Cadence, which is the speed at which you are pedaling.
- To the right, you'll see Resistance. This is controlled by the orange knob underneath the handlebars. If you turn the knob to the left, you will feel less pressure, and the pedaling will become easier. When you turn it to the right, the pedaling will get tougher—just as if you were cycling up a hill. The Resistance number on the screen will go higher the more you turn the knob to the right.
- Finally, the omnipresent number at the center of your screen will show your Output. This number is calculated using the combination of your Cadence and Resistance. In my opinion, this represents the "Holy Grail" of Peloton because it's a good indicator of how much effort you have put in on your ride. Your total Output is shown in kilojoules (kj), which is another way of saying one thousand joules. A joule is one-watt in one second. So, for example, one joule of energy can light a one watt light bulb for one second. That might not sound like much, but when you add it all up, the energy you burn can be quite astounding!

Unless it's your thing, I wouldn't get hung up on complex calculations. Suffice to say, your effort is measured by how hard you're working during a ride and for how long you've been working.

One quirk: Sometimes the Output on the bottom is off from the Output shown on the Leaderboard. Don't worry! That's only because it takes longer for the system to update the metrics on the Leaderboard.

In addition, if you have a heart monitor, those metrics will also appear on the left side of the screen.

The Leaderboard is where the rubber hits the road. It's here where you can make your ride competitive—if you like—and see how you measure up against real people. (For folks who are not competitive, or find this intimidating or annoying, you can easily swipe it away with a right finger movement on the screen.)

I think engaging with the Leaderboard can be more fun if you understand what the numbers mean.

The first thing you will want to do is find your username. Let's assume you have never taken a ride and therefore have no Personal Record (PR) for this type of class or scenic ride. That's okay! The status bar not only shows your username, but the number to the left will show your position on the ride. At the top of the Leaderboard, you'll see that you have two choices: "All Time" and "Here Now."

If you tap on All Time, your position number will display where you are relative to everyone who has ever taken that ride. If you tap on Here Now, you'll see what

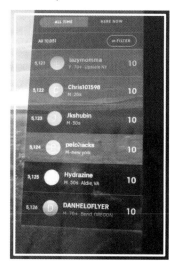

your position is against people presently riding. You will also notice a "Filter" button. With this choice, you can literally filter it down to certain people you are following; this means you can tell how you're doing compared to just those people.

When you start riding, you should see a circle around your avatar. This is actually a clock. It becomes shaded to indicate how much time has elapsed. This is so, when you compare yourself to others on the same ride, you can tell if they started before you did.

Below your username you'll see information about you including your sex, your age, and your location label. This information is collected from your Peloton profile. You can choose to show or hide this information, as you like, through your Peloton preferences.

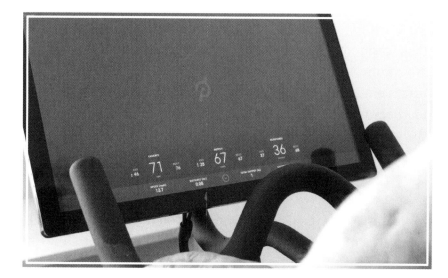

To the right on the Leaderboard is your Output number, which corresponds to the Output number that displayed on the bottom of the screen between Cadence and Resistance. The Output number determines your rank on the leaderboard.

If you have previously taken a similar ride, the leaderboard will also show your Personal Record (PR) either above the main status bar, or right below it. If, for instance, you took a twenty-minute beginner class, it will show your personal record in parentheses next to the type of class you took. It will also give you, to the far right, a pacing number indicating what you did in the class in which you achieved your Personal Record. In this way, you can compare that best with how you're doing in the ride you're currently on. If you are not keeping up to the pace of your PR, this information will go on top of your status bar. If you are doing better at this point in the ride, it will go below the status bar.

It takes some time to see how this all plays out when you are comparing yourself to others on the ride, especially if you didn't start at the same time. But I think you'll find—once you get into it a little bit—that it can be galvanizing and fun to compare yourself to others, and/or to try to match or exceed your personal best.

PELO TIP 20: SO, WHAT'S FTP?

In the next section of this book, I'll introduce you to something called *Power Zone Training*. But before you can use Power Zones, you will need to assess what you are capable of in a twenty-minute ride. This is referred to as your twenty-minute average. By testing yourself in a twenty-minute period of time, you will be able to calculate your FTP. Confused yet? Wondering why this is a good thing? Stay with me.

Before you take this twenty-minute test, I highly recommend that you do some really good stretch exercises, easily found on the Peloton App. Then you should hop on the bike and do something called the "10 Min FTP Warm Up Ride." To find this class, tap on "Programs" on the bottom tool bar of your screen. Under training programs, tap "Discover Your Power Zones." In that grouping you will find the "10 Min FTP Warm Up Ride."

So enough suspense. What's FTP?

FTP stands for Functional Threshold Power. The warm-up ride I'm recommending here prepares you for the intensity of finding what your personal threshold is. So, psych yourself up for an intense half hour where you will push yourself to the limit. Directly after completing the warm-up, go back to the "Programs" tab on the bottom tool bar. Once again, tap "Discover Your Power Zones." There you will see the

"20 Minute Test Ride." Now tap that and follow the instructions from your leader. As always, make sure you are hydrated and have a towel at the ready!

At the end of your ride, your twenty-minute average FTP output will be displayed on your ride recap. Your FTP will be important as you move into Power Zone Training.

PELO TIP 21: POWER ZONES

Now to Power Zones! Power Zone training is aimed at challenging you to improve your strength and endurance. There are seven Power Zones presented on a continuum from "Very Easy" to "Max Effort." Each Power Zone represents a target output range customized for each rider. In my household, my seven zones are different from my wife's, and our sons all have different zones based on their individual outputs. During a Power Zone Ride, you will hear your instructor call out a specific Zone, which you will then endeavor to achieve. Other riders on the Leaderboard will be at their own Output levels, but you and they will be in the same Zones. See the difference? The purpose of the zone system is to see if you can improve over time, by competing against others but keeping your progress customized to you.

To use Power Zones, you will first need to figure out your average output during a twenty-minute ride. Once you have that average, you can calculate your FTP and, from there, figure out your target output for each of the seven zones.

Don't worry! It sounds more complicated than it is. Here are the steps that Peloton recommends:

1. Take the "10 Min FTP Warm Up Ride," which, as stated above, is found in the "Power Zone Program."
2. Immediately afterward, complete a "20 Min FTP Test Ride," also in the "Power Zone Program."
3. When you complete your ride, seek your twenty-minute average on the ride recap screen.

To learn more, go to your home screen and tap on the three dots in the lower right-hand corner. On the pop-up menu, tap "Profile Settings." Then, under "Preferences," scroll down until you find "Display Power Zones" and tap on it. Under "Power Zones FTP," choose "Custom Value." There you will see a pop-up keyboard. Now enter your best average output over twenty minutes to set your Functional Threshold Power (FTP). And when you're finished, tap "OK."

The good news is that you don't have to do the math. The bike's computer does all of that for you. And once you've taken these steps, Power Zones will show up on your display for every ride. If you like, you can take the "20 Min FTP Test" ride at a later date to see if your twenty-minute average output has increased. You can then enter the new numbers to update your output ranges.

On all successive rides, you will see a bar below your metrics. It lights up in different colors as your output goes up and down. The colors correspond to your power ranges and target output ranges.

To review, these are the seven Power Zones:

Zone 1 **Very Easy**	<55% of FTP Characterized as warm-up or recovery
Zone 2 **Moderate**	56-75% of FTP Characterized as a comfortable, long ride
Zone 3 **Sustainable**	76-90% of FTP Should be sustainable for over an hour
Zone 4 **Challenging**	91-105% of FTP Sustainable for up to an hour
Zone 5 **Hard**	106-120% of FTP Sustainable for 10–15 minutes at most
Zone 6 **Very Hard**	121-150% of FTP Sustainable for 30 seconds to 3–5 min. max.
Zone 7 **Max Effort**	>151% of FTP Sustainable for only a few seconds

PELO TIP 22: CUSTOM AUDIO

Let's face it: some days you'll need the encouragement of an instructor to help you get through the ride, but other times you want something else, like music, perhaps. But what are riders to do if they prefer a musical accompaniment to their workout?

In the spring of 2019, Peloton made an effort to address this situation in many of their on-demand classes and allow for a musical option. Now, let me be clear from the outset: Peloton's solution is still far from perfect. However, it *is* a first step in allowing you some control when it comes to deter-mining which audio element has the higher volume: the instructor or the soundtrack.

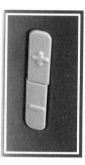

How do you adjust the volume-to-instructor ratio? The answer is *NOT* by using the on-screen volume control. Instead, you'll need to press the volume buttons on the right side of the back of the tablet.

When you do this, a pop-up menu will appear on your screen. (You might need to keep your finger on the volume control because it quickly disappears.) This pop-up menu displays three choices from left to right: more music, original mix, and more instructor. Above these boxes, you will find a volume bar; slide it right to increase the volume of that audio element, and left to decrease it.

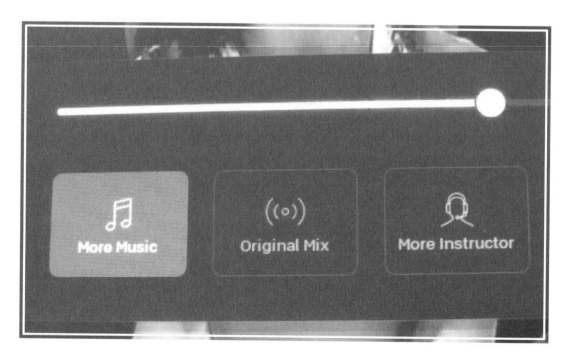

To be clear, these volume controls do not give you the ability to eliminate either the instructor or music completely, but you can still go a long way toward emphasizing the one you want to hear. Further, this feature works with both the built-in speakers and headphones. And if you change your mind about the audio mix and want to reset things, simply tap the volume buttons again until your mix is recalibrated.

Probably the number one question people ask at this point is "What about *my* music?"

Well, if the music Peloton plays is not to your liking—and you'd prefer to pedal to something else entirely—there's a solution, albeit an imperfect one.

If you want to listen to your own music, slide the volume bar all the way to the left and play your personal music on a Bluetooth device. Obviously, you won't hear the instructor in this scenario, but you will still have the visual cues on the screen to guide you toward reaching the desired metrics for your ride. For many riders who want to hear their own custom playlist during their workout, this trade-off is more than worth it.

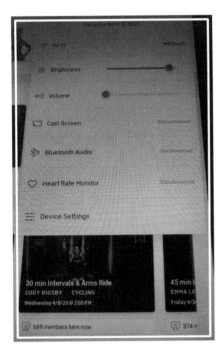

Personally, I go along with the musical choices that the instructors choose. Using Peloton's built-in filters, I have some choice of music genre or even particular artists and decades. I also like that I can change the ratio of music during the on-demand rides by pressing volume control on the back of the touch screen.

But there's one genre of music where I put my foot down—and not in a good way! I just can't stand the cheesy electronic music that accompanies the scenic rides. It's so off-putting, and in my opinion it seems utterly incompatible with the video element when you're riding the streets of Paris or traveling down a country road in New England.

So before I start a scenic ride, my solution is to go to the upper right-hand corner of the touch screen and tap "Settings." Then I scroll down the menu until I see volume. I slide the bar all the way to the left, which essentially makes it mute. Then I go to the music library on my phone, find a nice playlist I've created for the ride, and synch it to a Bluetooth speaker in my workout room. Then I get on the bike and enjoy the high-quality music playing from the speaker, which is a more appropriate playlist for my workout. It's total bliss!

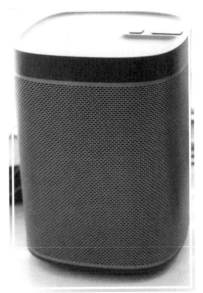

PELO TIP 23: CLOSED CAPTIONS

Studies have been done on the effects of subtitles in movies on an audience. These studies reveal a variety of responses. While some find it distracting to see subtitles, others find that they understand the dialogue, characters, and story arc much better when they can read the lines being spoken.

Everybody's brain works differently, and I imagine it is no different when you are watching an instructor in an exercise class.

Personally, I like doing the workouts with the closed captions on, using my tablet or phone. (Not so much on the bike, when it competes with other metrics that are showing up on the touch screen.) The reason I like it for the off-the-bike workouts is because the speakers on my phone and iPad are not ideal, and when the balance of music to voice is off, closed captioning helps me to see something I might have missed via the audio. This is especially helpful during a complicated exercise during which I need to concentrate (and/or when the tablet or phone is not necessarily as close as the touch screen on the bike).

To turn the closed caption function on, tap on a class that you want to take. A box will pop up that gives you a preview of the class you are about to take, including the rating, level of difficulty, the equipment you will need, the music that will be featured by artist and track, and the class plan. There is also a brief description of the class. Directly below that description is the "Closed Caption" box. Tap on it to indicate you want to have subtitles and then tap the red "Start" tab. As soon as the instructor starts talking, you should be able to see the closed captions. When you are finished with the workout, remember to go back in and tap the closed caption box again to turn it off for the next time (so that it doesn't remain on when you next use your bike).

PELO TIP 24: TARGET METRICS

One of the neat things about Peloton is that no two instructors or classes are exactly the same. You can use this uniqueness to customize your own workouts as you move closer and closer toward meeting your fitness goals. However, for some riders, the sheer variety of choices available can be daunting. For example, sometimes you know which types of training goals you want to achieve, but you don't know which class(es) will help you get there. The good news is that Peloton offers significant help when it comes to determining which classes are right for you. Many on-demand rides allow you to preview the scope of Resistance and Cadence that will be featured in that particular ride. You access this information by selecting a class and tapping it once. You will then see the preview pane. In this pane, you can scroll down to see the metrics (and even music) that will be in that ride. This preview can allow you to determine beforehand if a ride's target metrics are going to be in sync with what you're shooting for.

Another word about target metrics: Once you start a ride, you may occasionally space out and fail to hear what an instructor just said about increasing or decreasing the Resistance or Cadence. (Goodness knows, it's happened to me a number of times!) But if this happens, don't worry! Peloton has you covered. Ranges will be displayed on the screen directly above the resistance, output, and cadence you are currently achieving. If you miss a verbal adjustment from the instructor, you're bound to see it reflected here, as well.

PELO TIP 25: ON THE CHEAP

I've struggled with where to put this tip—or if I should even include it—but I think it's vital to speak to this issue somewhere because it's relevant to so many riders and potential riders.

Let's just say you don't want to invest the two thousand-plus dollars for the Peloton Bike or commit to the first-year subscription of forty dollars per month. What are your options? Well, what some people have done is to find a way to simulate the experience. For example, you could get a decent spin bike for around three hundred dollars. Some of these even come with the essential resistance knob. Then you could subscribe to the Peloton App for a price of twenty dollars per month, something the company offers for people who don't own the Peloton Bike. You get the same terrific classes, but just not on a fancy Peloton Touch Screen. You would want to get a tablet or phone holder that is attached to the handlebars of your spin bike. And you would also want to get a separate cadence monitor. If you have a smart TV in the room where you're riding, you could even cast the particular class onto the bigger screen.

Obviously, this solution isn't the same as purchasing a real Peloton Bike. However, because Peloton offers the app in anticipation that many people are going to do this, I don't think anyone ought to feel it qualifies as "cheating." For example, some people might be considering making the purchase of a Peloton Bike, but before they do, they want to ensure that it's the kind of exercise they will enjoy and stick with. (This might be someone who has never ridden any kind of exercise bike before.) For these folks, I think that using the app can be a great way of gauging their own response to a bike before making a big purchase. And for folks who simply aren't going to have the true Peloton Bike within their budget for the foreseeable future, this method can be an acceptable long-term work-around.

PELO TIP 26: JAILBREAKING

Jailbreaking is another controversial topic. In the interest of full disclosure, I should note that I have not done this, but many Peloton users have. Rather than watching the workout videos, live classes, and scenic rides with prerecorded music (for the monthly fee that Peloton charges), some users have taken to jailbreaking their Pelotons. This involves hacking into the Peloton and using it to view whatever content you like, free from the Peloton subscription service.

The company warns explicitly against doing this, and it will certainly take your tablet out of warranty. Nonetheless, many Peloton jailbreakers are rooting the Android-based tablet in order to access apps like Netflix and Spotify during their rides.

If you're a self-styled hacker and this type of thing appeals to you, there are instructions available on the Internet showing you how to do it. But please let me be very clear: you do so at your own peril. Your bike is a big investment. When you take it out of warranty, you are putting that investment at risk.

Personally, jailbreaking is just not my thing. I'm here for the full workout experience. But I won't judge you if you feel you would be most satisfied by using your Peloton in a different way.

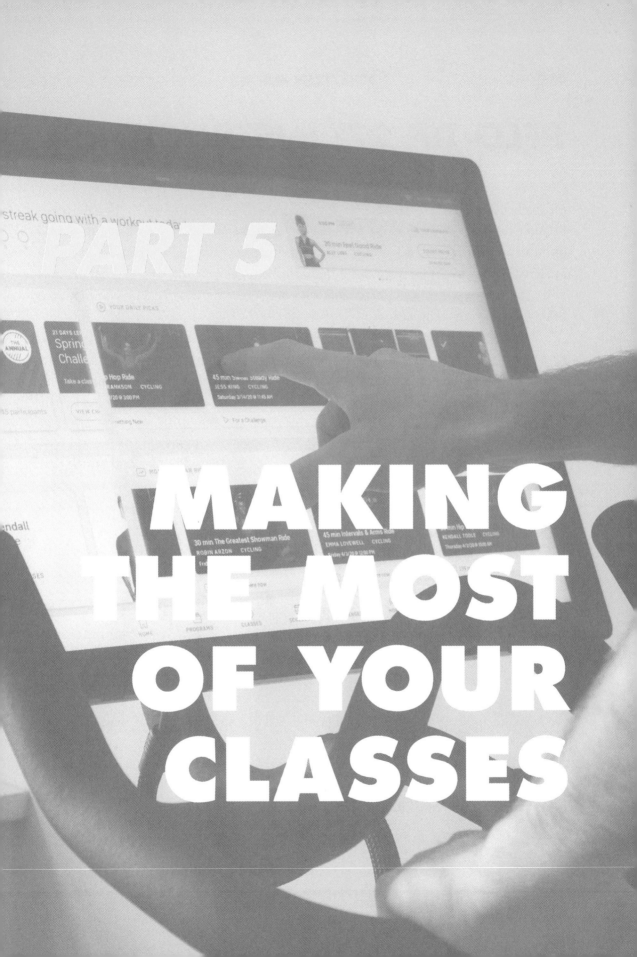

PART 5

MAKING THE MOST OF YOUR CLASSES

PELO TIP 27: INSTRUCTORS

Obviously, your choice of Peloton instructor is going to be very subjective. I can't recommend specific instructors to you, because I don't know what your personal preferences are (or if you even have them). You may find that you have no strong opinion on instructors, or you may find that some are excellent for you, while others are lousy. (It's okay! They won't be in the same room as you and won't take it personally.) You may settle on one instructor who becomes your favorite, or you may find that you enjoy constant variation.

My advice is to try a wide range of classes taught by different instructors as you first begin your Peloton journey. Each instructor is different and brings a unique approach to leading a workout. If you are new to this type of exercise, I suggest you go to the twenty-minute Beginner Rides ("Welcome to Peloton Cycling"). As I write this, there are eighteen classes offered in this program. I'm guessing that, over time, Peloton will add more. But for now, eighteen is more than enough to let you experience the wide variety of instructors and their approaches (not to mention their music selections). I encourage you to try all of them. See which ones fit. If you like, you can even go to the instructors' Facebook and/or Instagram pages to get to know them better.

When I was a beginner rider, I switched off every other ride, alternating between a scenic ride and an instructor-led class. In this way, I was able to keep it interesting and find the right amount of variation.

Also, as you get in better shape and become a more accomplished rider, you can expect your preferences to change. That's okay! An instructor who "did it for you" back in the day might no longer be the right fit as you evolve. Don't be surprised if this happens. (Again, your instructors won't take it personally because they won't know!)

Also, an interesting element of Peloton to keep in mind is that many instructors offer terrific off-the-bike workouts that can include yoga, stretching, running, and meditation classes. In conclusion, I encourage you to be "the Captain Kirk of Peloton." Explore the wide variety of people who are there to help you reach your fitness and wellness goals. Enjoy the journey!

PELO TIP 28: BOOKMARKING A FAVORITE CLASS

With so many choices of instructors, classes, and scenic rides, it can be challenging to remember all of your favorites. And nothing's more annoying than finding a class that feels perfect to do again in the future, but forgetting where on the system it's saved.

Peloton has a nice solution. You can bookmark and save your favorite classes to reride whenever the mood strikes you. To do this, simply click the ribbon at the top right of the class preview screen. This class will then be saved directly to your profile.

And to find all your previously saved items, go to "Classes" and tap on the ribbon icon in the upper left corner. This will take you to a menu of all your bookmarked classes.

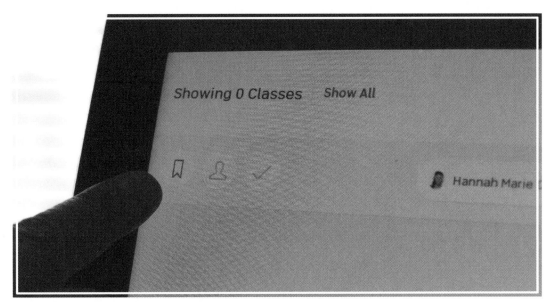

PELO TIP 29: LIVE VS. ON-DEMAND

Some Peloton riders really love the immediacy of the live ride. They thrive on the energy of the people in the studio, and on knowing that other riders all over the world are doing the same thing at the same time. These riders also love the occasional shout-out from the instructor for a milestone or great achievement. Finally, these are the kind of people who thrive on the discipline that is built with showing up for an appointment.

You may find that you are precisely this kind of rider!

When you sign up for a live ride, you will receive an alert in your email. And if you like, you can check in five minutes before the ride begins and observe the instructor chatting with the in-studio riders as they—and you—warm up. It's fun, and it gives you the sense that you are an actual part of a live event.

But what if you're **NOT** this kind of rider? What if an instructor somewhere halfway across the country acknowledging you is creepy and weird? What if the idea of keeping an appointment for a workout makes you feel an additional layer of stress in your already stressed-out workday?

If this is the case, Peloton has you covered here, too.

You're probably one of the many people who will love the huge selection of prerecorded, on-demand classes that you can start at any time. These classes can be engaged with at your leisure. An appointment running long or an unexpected interruption will be no big deal.

To each his own. Both approaches have something to offer. (And if you want to get really creative, you can always alternate between live and prerecorded classes.)

PELO TIP 30: THE CENTURY RIDE

You'll hear Peloton enthusiasts talk about "the Century Ride." What is this? What do they mean?

No, it doesn't mean riding your bike for a hundred years (though that would be an accomplishment). In fact, the Century Ride is the milestone that you reach when completing your one-hundredth class ride.

If you meet this accomplishment during a live class, you might even get a shout-out from the instructor. After reaching this milestone, you will become eligible to receive a Peloton Century Shirt. Peloton usually sends an email within a week and gives you a special code to redeem your shirt. (Make sure you enter that code, because without it you will be charged a hefty price. You will also be expected to pay the shipping.) The Peloton Century Shirt is a fun way to brag to your friends, family, and other Peloton riders about your accomplishment. It can also be a great symbol for yourself of your remarkable personal accomplishment.

PELO TIP 31: RIDING IN TRIBES

"Tribes" is the word used to describe groups of Peloton riders who choose to bike together. (Or, that is to say, "virtually" together.)

While some riders prefer to ride in anonymity, others relish the social aspect that comes with belonging to a community and choose to engage with the aspects of the Peloton ride that can bring a feeling of community and group fun.

If you look at the Leaderboard during a group ride, you might notice different hashtags representing like-minded people, people of the same profession, or even those who like the same television program. These like-minded riders bond and decide to ride at the same time and usually connect on social media outside of the ride. We call them tribes. It can feel a little strange when explained like this, but during a ride you'll see that feeling out others in your community (practically any sort of community) can come naturally and be a whole lot of fun.

I think that the tribes phenomenon just goes to prove how working out on a Peloton Bike can be a very social activity. And knowing that you're pedaling away with other patent lawyers, dog lovers, or fans of *Battlestar Galactica* can be yet another way to motivate you to get in shape.

PELO TIP 32: MEET THE PELOTONS

If you live in New York City (or are visiting), you may wish to take a live ride in the Peloton Studio itself. Talk about being in the room where it happens! You just might get to meet a favored instructor or someone like yourself who has fallen in love with the Peloton lifestyle.

So how does showing up in person actually work? Through the website (https://

studio.onepeloton.com), you will have to pay a fee and make a reservation in advance to get one of the coveted spots—so you can't just show up—but included in your reservation will be refreshments and the use of the showers. And if you don't have your own shoes with you, they will lend you a pair.

When showing up for a live ride, it is generally a good idea to know things like your seat height and depth, and handlebar height, as well as your login username and password. This will allow you to "hit the ride running," so to speak, when it's time to go.

PELO TIP 33: SWIPE AWAY

Some days, you're going to find that you just don't feel like a peak performer. That's okay. It happens to everybody. On these days, it can feel like you showed up, and they should give you a medal just for that!

In my case, on the mornings when I work out before going to work, I often feel like the ride will go on forever. I'm cranky and tired, and just staying on the bike feels like a supreme effort. Psychologically, it helps me not to know how much time I have remaining. So rather than not look at the screen, I tap the timer at the top left of the touch screen to remove the timer. Likewise, that Leaderboard. There are days when I am deflated because no matter what, I can't muster the strength to beat anybody, let alone my own personal record. Double tap on the middle of the screen. Poof. It is gone. But the video is still there and I can live with that. (Double-tap again and it all comes back.)

The disappearing metrics are especially nice when you do a scenic ride. All you see are those beautiful vistas. It can lift your spirits and get you through the ride, and you're not worried about comparing yourself to how you did that one time when you'd just had ten hours of sleep and a pep talk.

In conclusion, the social and performance-tracking elements of the Peloton experience can be motivating and exciting . . . but when they become the opposite of those things—and you feel like just completing the ride is the biggest "win" you can realistically hope for—then don't be afraid to just turn them off and be in your own headspace. Remember, the Peloton is there to help *you* meet *your* fitness goals. It's great that it can do that by being a social entity. However, if you just need it to be quiet for a while—and not bother you with comparisons and personal bests—that's okay, too!

PELO TIP 34: VIDEO CHATS

There is a video camera on your Peloton Bike monitor. And it is pointed at **you**. (As creepy as that may sound, there is no cause for concern. The Peloton instructor cannot see you without your permission, and there are—to my knowledge—no cases of Peloton cameras being hacked and videos of people working out captured without their permission.) The camera is there to allow you to have in-class video chats with instructors and friends—if that's something you want to do.

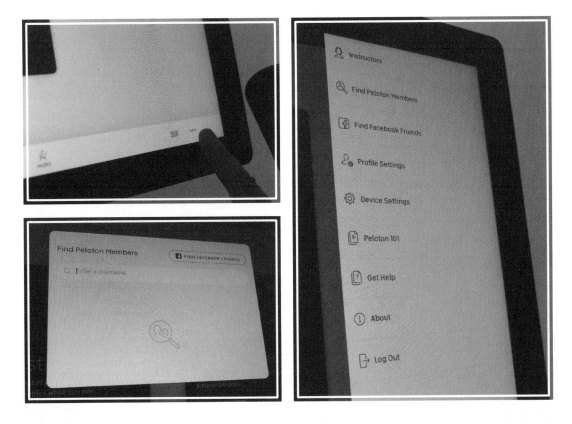

Some people find this option motivating; they think of it as just another way to be part of a large community. Others like the camera because it connects to the idea of "misery loves company." They think: "If I am going to suffer during my workout, at least I want to suffer with a friend."

To activate the camera function that can connect you with other riders, you'll first need to be following the other person, and vice versa. This is similar to how you follow someone on any sort of social network. Then, on the Leaderboard, you click on the user's name. You will then see an option to start a video chat. Once you send the chat request, the other person will have to accept for the chat to go live. If and when they do, a small pop-up box with audio/video will then appear on the screen, allowing you to see each other. You can mute the other person at any time and also control the volume on the bar below the video screen. Now you are ready for your close-up. (Just make sure you have your clothes on!)

PELO TIP 35: DELETING A CLASS

I'm a stickler for accuracy and keeping my metrics honest and true. But let's say that one day I break my cardinal rule and get off the bike to answer a phone call (and the class keeps going without me). Now, I don't want the tablet to keep that class in my personal history. So what do I do? I delete it. And if you find yourself in this situation, you can do the very same thing.

To delete a class, simply tap on your profile name on the lower left-hand corner, then tap on "Workout History" on the left. In the middle pane, make sure the class you wish to remove is highlighted. On the larger, right-hand pane, you will see the metrics of that class. Scroll all the way down to the end. At the very bottom, on the left side, you will see "Delete Workout" in red. Tap there and then tap again to confirm.

Boom! Now it's like that phone call never happened.

PELO TIP 36: MAINTENANCE OF YOUR BIKE

As with any big investment, you'll obviously want to take care of your Peloton Bike. Yet because the bikes are a very new technology, there's still some question about what good maintenance can or can't do.

To put it frankly, there is no certainty regarding how long these bikes can last; there is a wide range of stories of people having problems—from faulty touch screens to threads on a pedal messing up their rides—but we don't know how many of these examples were caused by user error, and/or to what extent they could have been prevented if more care had been taken.

But just because there are many unknowns when it comes to the life of a Peloton Bike, that doesn't mean that we can't move forward using good old common sense.

As with any other appliance or piece of large equipment, taking care of your Peloton Bike shows every sign of being able to mitigate unnecessary problems down the road. The first step in good care is simply cleaning the bike, which Peloton suggests doing after every ride.

When cleaning the touch screen, it is advised that you first shut down the tablet using the power button in the back. To clean the screen, wipe it down with a glass cleaner or a microfiber cloth. Do not use Clorox wipes or similar cloths and do not use any harsh chemicals when cleaning the screen.

When it comes to cleaning the frame, use a gentle cleanser or disinfectant wipes. Do not use soap and water. Never spray anything directly on the bike. Dry the bike thoroughly after cleaning.

It is recommended that every three to five rides you also make sure the seat is parallel to the ground. This is not a cleaning step per se, but more of a maintenance step. Your delivery people should have given you some tools for the bike before they left. Use the wrench they left to tighten the seat, fixing nuts on both sides. You should then use the 4mm Allen wrench to tighten any loose screws attaching your cleats to your cycling shoes.

Every fifteen to twenty rides, Peloton recommends that you press down on the resistance knob while pedaling slowly. The flywheel should come to a complete stop immediately. If it does not, contact Peloton Support and let them know. They can take steps to help you fix this problem with the knob.

By keeping your bike clean and taking the small steps recommended for general maintenance, you can help ensure your bike has the best possible chance of lasting long into the future.

PELO TIP 37: THE GROOVE RIDE

Let's get this party started!

So let's say you've had the bike a little while, and you are feeling good about your progress. You can handle a lot of what the instructors are shouting out regarding speed, pressure on your pedal, and getting up and out of your saddle. Now, every so often, you feel like you want to do more than just up your cadence, raise your resistance, and get off your seat for more than thirty seconds. When these feelings arise, you might want to consider the "Groove Ride" classes offered by some of the Peloton instructors.

In these challenging classes, you will be encouraged to execute choreographed movements to the beat of the music in the background. Specifically, you will be incorporating something called "tap backs"—a sort of standing ab crunch—which you do off the saddle, slowly curling the hips back, moving up, down, and to the sides. You will also learn "bike pushups," which have you bending the elbows so that your torso comes forward to the handlebars, then straightening your arms out again—all while pedaling. I kid you not!

As you might imagine, it's quite a workout. It's also a heck of a lot of fun.

Some people get so caught up in this big dance party, they don't realize how high their outputs are. In my experience, you're likely to do a double take when you finally do look at your metrics. You may be having so much fun that you haven't noticed how hard you've been working. The Groove Ride is a challenging workout, but do check it out when you are ready. If you're feeling ready to push yourself, there's no time like the present.

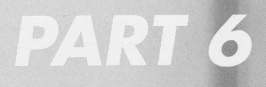

PART 6

PELOTON OUT IN THE WORLD

PELO TIP 38: SALES ALERTS

Past is not necessarily prologue when it comes to Peloton pricing dynamics. As any smart consumer knows, there is no guarantee that a company will be consistent in its sales and marketing strategies over time, and Peloton is no exception. As of this writing, there seems to be a prevalent belief that the price of the basic bike and tablet is not going to go down. Think of it like other high-end products, such as those made by Apple. The quality stays high, but there are regular price increases.

Likewise, the monthly subscription costs are also not projected to creep down anytime soon. As an example, when I got my bike, the subscription was forty dollars per month, and I was locked in for a year. A couple of months later, there were advertisements running on my television saying that the monthly subscription now costs fifty-eight dollars per month. And who knows what will happen if competitors like NordicTrack or Fly Wheel encroach on Peloton's space. (I feel that could impact prices either way.)

Having said that, there are some sales that Peloton occasionally runs, and you should look out for them if you're interested in pulling the trigger. For example, the annual holiday sales event usually has a lower-priced package for the mat, shoes, headphones, and monitor. Further, the winter sales event gives you 30 percent off select apparel, including workout clothes and accessories. Simply get on the Peloton mailing list (https://www.onepeloton.com/company/contact) to learn about these and other offers.

There's no way to know for certain which way the pricing for Peloton products and services will go—and when—but by staying informed, you can be ready to take advantage of offers and act when the time is right.

PELO TIP 39: WHEN YOU TRAVEL

When I started riding my Peloton Bike, I got on a great streak, working out every single day. I felt good, and, not to be immodest, I was looking better than I had for a long while. But then I found out that I had a business trip coming up that I just couldn't miss. Of course, I could have ridden other bikes in a hotel gym during this trip, but I was worried about changing my routine.

As it turned out, I needn't have been so concerned.

A little research into the hotels in the city I was traveling to revealed that three of them offered Peloton Bikes for guests. I chose the hotel that boasted a stable of four Peloton Bikes—just in case there were going to be other obsessives like me in town at the same time. I also called ahead to ask what type of pedals the bikes had; I wanted to see if I needed to pack my Peloton shoes. As it turned out, they had toe cages, so sneakers would be adequate and I was good to go. I think there's good evidence that, going forward, more and more hotels are going to be standing ready to accommodate Peloton riders who want to keep up their workouts while traveling on business. Three years ago, Peloton formed a partnership with Marriott's Westin Hotels and Resorts, and they are looking to do more.

And if you find yourself in an area that doesn't yet have Peloton Bikes, you can do the next best thing and use the Peloton app for all the great exercises offered for those without a bike, including outside activities.

As a final note, let me say that I've personally found that when I return home from a business trip, the Peloton Bike does wonders for helping to correct my jet lag!

PELO TIP 40: WHEN YOU DON'T TRAVEL

One reason I think a Peloton Bike is such an excellent investment is all the workout options it gives you—all of which are doable from the safety and security of your own home. Sometimes the benefits of Peloton classes can extend beyond just eliminating the hassle of physically traveling to and from the gym. Sometimes there can be important reasons to stay home!

You may have children to watch or important situations to monitor. And as the coronavirus pandemic of 2020 made clear, there can be certain times when the idea of being in a close-quarters gym with a bunch of sweaty strangers is not an appealing idea for a whole host of reasons, or is not even legally allowed.

If you're considering buying a Peloton Bike, but see yourself as a more social, "out-in-the-world" person when it comes to exercising, you may still want to consider the purchase. In the short term, if your car has a flat and you suddenly can't drive to the gym, or the weather is too lousy to go for an outdoor ride, the Peloton is an excellent fallback. And if something more serious happens—from a viral outbreak, to an outbreak of crime or unrest in your neighborhood, to something completely unforeseen—having the Peloton lets you know that you always have options.

PELO TIP 41: HOW TO SCREENCAST FROM BIKE TO TV

Let's say that you want to do some exercises off the bike—say, on a mat that's in the same room. One way some ambitious riders accomplish this is to remove the tablet from the bike and direct the screen to where they can see it on the mat. Because this involves first removing the cables at the back of the tablet and then using Allen and crescent wrenches (first taking off the plastic end caps) to remove the bolt connecting the tablet to the bike, I don't recommend this approach for the general Peloton rider. (Though it *is* possible to do.) There is always the potential to damage the tablet in some way, and even if you really know what you are doing, it can be time-consuming and cumbersome—which might be a deterrent from getting to your exercise at all.

The good news is that Peloton offers you a wireless alternative to moving the tablet. Peloton has anticipated that you may want to see your programs on a big television screen, or maybe you'll want to do off-bike exercises in a room other than the one where your bike is set up. This is called "screen casting." To use this feature, it is required that you have a device or a Smart TV that supports Miracast. (Please note that the Peloton tablet does not support Apple airplay or Chromecast. Devices that generally work are the Amazon Fire TV Stick and most of the new Roku devices.)

Before you start setting up your wireless option, make sure that the television and/or device is turned on and then check that your Wi-Fi is on, even if you use Ethernet. On the upper right-hand corner of your Peloton tablet, you'll tap "Settings." Then you'll tap "Cast Screen." A list will then populate on the "Available Devices." Find your device or TV and tap "Connect." On the television, you should be able to see the same thing that is displayed on the screen of your tablet.

If you don't have the right device or Smart TV, or your Wi-Fi doesn't work in the room where the bike is set up, try using another tablet, like an iPad, or a phone to play exercises on the Peloton app. It's a decent work-around to play your off-the-bike exercises. As with any amount of technical equipment setup, there are bound to be glitches and hiccups. However, most users with the right equipment are able to successfully use this option, and I hope that you can, too!

PELO TIP 42: POWERING YOUR DEVICE

Not to belabor the obvious, but if you have moved your bike or forgotten how the delivery people fired up your bike, you'll need to remember how to power it up. The power jack is located at the very back of the bike. Plug the power cord into the jack, and then—to play it safe—plug the other end into a surge protector. (Just as you would with any valuable piece of electronic equipment, I think it's important to surge-protect your Peloton.)

The power button that actually turns on the bike is located on the back of the tablet. Hold it for two seconds to power on.

Depending on the settings on your touch screen, the bike will "sleep" after five minutes of inactivity. To wake it, simply tap on the screen or press the power button. To power down, hold the button for two seconds. On the screen you will see a pop-up box. When it appears, simply tap "Shut Down."

PELO TIP 43: ETHERNET

Suppose you take a Peloton live class and it freezes! (Or, just as bad, it jumps, delays, or skips.) Generally speaking, this means you have a streaming issue. This may be because your modem is not close to where the bike is set up. There may be an interference issue with the Wi-Fi signal to the Peloton. You could try changing the channels on your Wi-Fi network, found in your router settings. The best solution might just be to streamline through an Ethernet cable.

On the back of the tablet is an Ethernet port, which allows you to connect to a wired network. Connect an Ethernet cable to the port and the other end to a wall jack or router. You will then be automatically connected to the network.

PELO TIP 44: WI-FI

Connecting to Wi-Fi on your Peloton Bike should be easy and straightforward.

To connect to Wi-Fi, tap on settings on the upper right-hand corner of the Peloton screen. Then tap on "Wi-Fi Network." Find your network name and tap on it. If your network is secured, you will be asked for your password. Enter it and then tap "Connect."

PELO TIP 45: LOGGING IN

When you first purchased your Peloton Bike, you were issued a subscription activation key (or you supplied Peloton with your log in information). When your bike is delivered and you log in for the first time, you will be asked for this information. Once activated, that information will forevermore be associated with your bike, and you'll then be able to access all subscription content. So make sure to remember your activation key and/or login information as you prepare to set up the bike!

PELO TIP 46: OTHER USERS

If other riders are going to be taking your Peloton Bike for a spin, you'll want them to set up their own profiles. The biggest reason for doing this is that you don't want their rides to screw up your personal metrics and ride history.

To set up other users, tap the menu icon on the lower left-hand corner of the touch screen. Then tap "Switch Rider." Tap "Manage Riders." Then tap "Add A Rider."

Your additional user can now log in with his or her Peloton account or set up a new one.

It's very easy to do, and you'll be glad you did it!

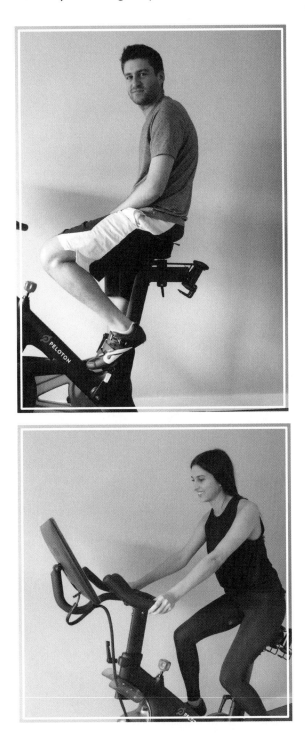

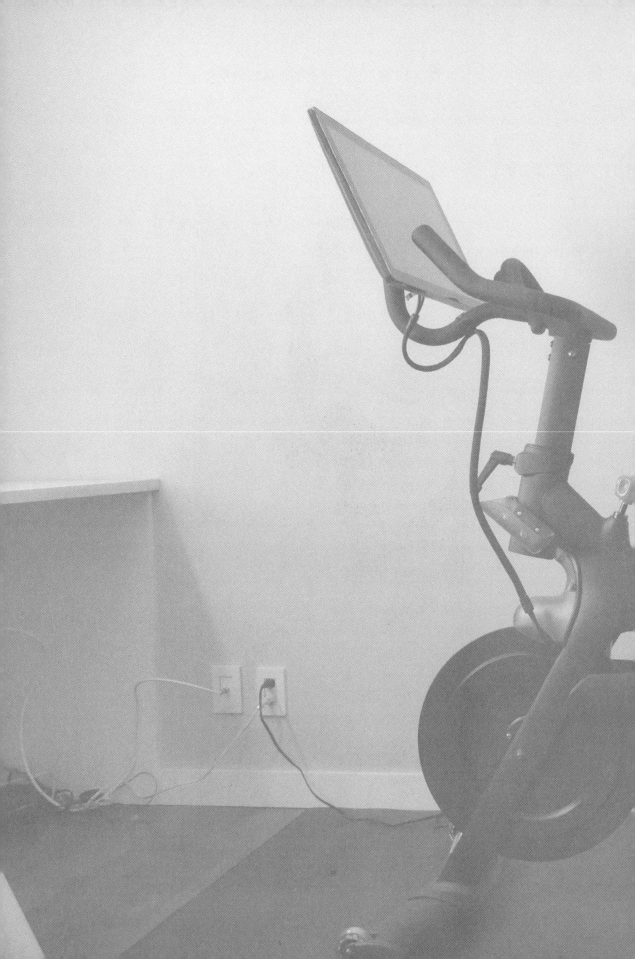

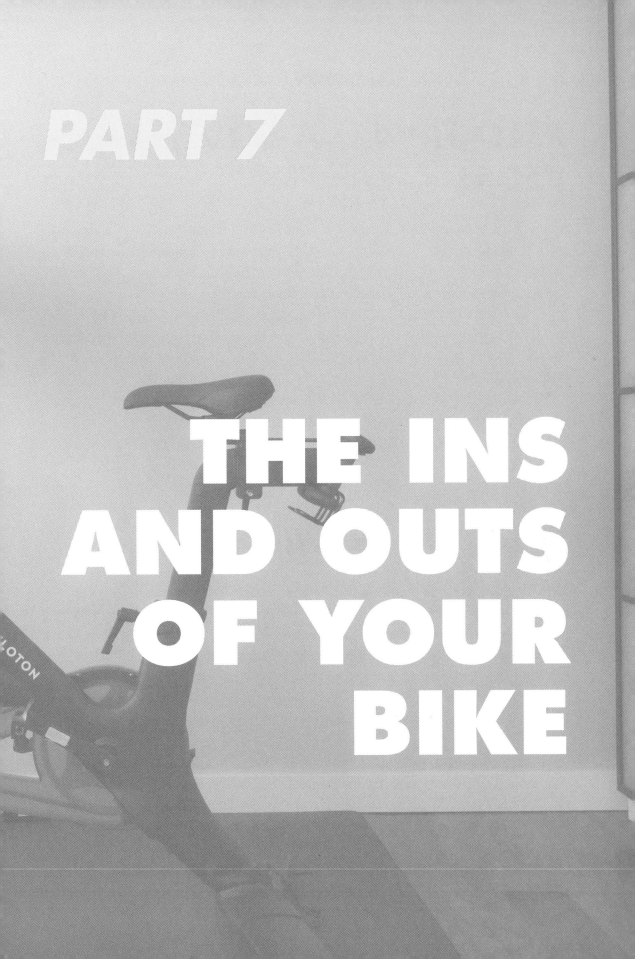

PART 7

THE INS AND OUTS OF YOUR BIKE

PELO TIP 47: A SQUEAKING PEDAL

Squeaks are a fairly common problem reported by Peloton riders. They especially seem to occur in exercise outings in which riders are prompted to get out of the saddle. Luckily, squeaks typically don't indicate that anything serious is wrong with the bike, but they sure can be annoying for the riders!

One of the most frequent causes of squeaks is your shoes. This has to do with the pedal rubbing against the shoe clip. If you think you're hearing a shoe-related squeak, you can purchase some dry lubricant aerosol and spray it on the cleat on the bottom of the shoe.

If you're hearing a squeak with an undetermined source, you'll want to first make sure the screws on the cleats and the pedal are tight.

If the problem still persists, you might want to try recording the problem and sending it to Peloton Support. They will be able to use your video to determine if it is a more serious problem and help you arrive at a good solution.

PELO TIP 48: HIIT RIDES

High-Intensity Interval Training (HIIT) is a cardiovascular exercise in which you perform short periods of intense anaerobic exercise, followed by less intense recovery periods. Typically, these exercises last thirty minutes, but times can sometimes vary.

HIIT training is very efficient for people who don't have a lot of time to work out but still want to see results. Physiologists agree that the reason this type of training can be effective is that it uses the body's reserves of energy. After a strenuous workout like this, your metabolism stays elevated and continues to burn calories long after the exercise.

Let me be up front about it: The Peloton HIIT classes will definitely challenge you. Talk about no pain/no gain! In thirty minutes or less, you'll get terrific fat-burning exercise, but it will certainly not be easy. On the other hand, if they're what you're looking for, don't let me scare you off. These bursts of high-intensity exercise, followed by varying periods of low-intensity active rest, can provide riders with motivation and fun—not to mention the confidence that you're going to be getting an excellent workout.

I definitely recommend starting with the ten-minute warm-ups. Peloton offers a lot of variety when it comes to the warm-up HIIT classes you can take. Play around with them to find the one that's right for you.

If you are away from your bike, you can also find excellent HIIT workouts on "Beyond the Ride" on your Peloton app. Here, I recommend starting with the five-minute beginner HIIT and then advancing to the fifteen-minute advanced HIIT.

HIIT may not be your thing—and it may never be your thing—and that's totally fine. However, I recommend trying it at least once. You may discover you like high-intensity workouts, and/or you may decide that they can be an option to enjoy occasionally (such as on a day when you're overscheduled, and the sixty minutes you set aside for working out just got cut to twenty).

PELO TIP 49: TABATA

Within the HIIT family is something referred to as the Tabata Protocol. Originated by a Japanese scientist named Dr. Izum Tabata in the early 1990s, this high-intensity interval training consists of eight sets of fast exercises, each performed for twenty seconds, followed by brief rests of ten seconds.

Studies have shown that Tabata workouts can improve aerobic fitness. In addition to causing the heart to pump faster, the exercise builds endurance and muscle. (When I do one, I swear I can almost see the calories burn off!)

Peloton offers Tabata rides as an option for those looking to see big results quickly but admittedly acknowledges that this is not a ride for beginners. Instead, Peloton promotes the Tabata rides as a way to break the repetition of other workouts you may be doing and urges you to "shock your body and see change."

Again, they're not for everybody, but if you feel like maybe your body needs a shock, Tabata is the way to go!

PELO TIP 50: APPLE HEALTH DATA

We live in a world in which technological advancements that allow us to do exciting new things are coming at us thick and fast; it seems that nowhere is this truer than

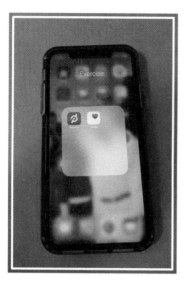

when it comes to tracking our health. Smartphones and smartwatches have the ability to monitor your daily activity (from steps taken to hours slept), storing it away so you can analyze it and sometimes fret about it.

It is both a blessing and a curse, but I think it's safe to say it is here to stay.

One problem we can encounter, however, is that our devices and apps don't always talk to each other. If you're a person who lives "between different brands," it can prove difficult to reconcile the data from all the competing tech companies. You will find that this tension is a part of Peloton ownership, as well.

From time to time, Peloton updates their software. One of their recent—and long-requested—feature updates literally happened while I was writing this Pelo Tip! (Talk about timely.) At this rate, I'm thinking there could be a whole new update by the time I get to the end of this paragraph. I'm sort of kidding, but sort of not.

Suffice it to say, Peloton is always working to make it easier to sync your workouts and ride history with recordings of other daily activity, such as in your Apple Health app. Peloton will even pull in your yoga workouts, which show up as "mindful minutes" in Apple Health. The metrics you will find are distance, heart rate, and other typically measured categories. (More advanced metrics like power data will require third-party tools.) Unfortunately, this capability is not yet extended to Android users. (But it may be by the time this book is published! I'm serious; new updates are happening all the time.)

To explore syncing your health data, in your Peloton app, start by tapping "More" on the lower right-hand corner of your screen. Then add on the Health pp (or Apple Watch) and sync. Then you can confirm that your Peloton data are showing up on your browser history under Activity/Workouts on the Apple Health app.

PELO TIP 51: FREE WEIGHTS

Just as it has in indoor cycling studios, performing upper body exercises has become all the rage on Peloton Bikes. I would be remiss if I didn't state up front that there are those who say that using free weights while pedaling is not only ineffective, but

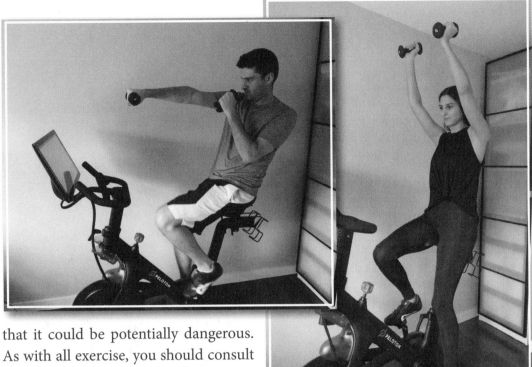

that it could be potentially dangerous. As with all exercise, you should consult with a doctor before you partake in any new type of ride. That being said, there are a lot of people who swear by the rides that incorporate free weights, so let's take a look and see if they could be right for you!

Let's start with how to "unsheathe" the weights. It is recommended that if you keep your free weights stored behind your seat, you start pedaling lightly, keeping an easy cadence and resistance, and then, carefully reaching behind you, take hold of the weights. Always maintain a straight posture. Once the weight is safely in your hand, there are plenty of options. You can do a repetition of fifteen bicep curls, reverse bicep curls, tricep pull downs—really, all the same stuff you do in your gym (or other spin classes) to help you get lean, toned arms.

Most of the rides available on your Peloton do not incorporate weights, but some do. I encourage you to experiment and try a ride with weights at least once. You'll discover whether or not you have a preference for them. Some Peloton users enjoy the rides with weights because—in my opinion—they feel like they are "killing two birds with one stone." Other riders may find the weights distracting or irritating during the ride and may prefer to let Peloton be just the cardio portion of their workouts and do different exercises for resistance.

To each his own; but I personally prefer to separate my cycling exercises from my weight training. For what it is worth, I **can** walk and chew gum at the same time. But hey, it's just not my thing!

PELO TIP 52: STANDING VS. SITTING

Some Peloton rides call for riders to stay seated, and others require riders (at least for portions of the ride) to stand. Yet within the Peloton community, you will find that there is also a stark divide on this issue. Some riders would prefer to stand as much as possible, and others, to sit.

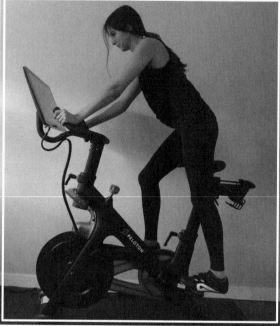

The reason that many riders like to stand is to increase the cardio benefits of riding their bike. Not only do you increase your heart rate when you stand, but standing can give a break to your legs (which might have gotten tired during the sitting portion of the exercise). Furthermore, people who have lower back pain swear that standing brings them relief.

During most rides, it will be a restricted amount of time for which you are standing. However, you may find yourself falling into the camp of people who like to stand as much as possible during the workout.

It is really important to take your resistance up during a standing portion, which will make each stride more like stepping on a physical stair; otherwise, it will be much harder on your legs. Remember: **the handlebars are just for balance**. Don't rely on them to support yourself.

When you go into a stand, slide your hands up a bit from where they were initially when you were in a sitting position. Don't go too far over/forward when you stand. Your hips should be low and still positioned over the saddle.

Work on your core strength—the series of muscles in your abdomen—if you feel you need to be stronger before doing the standing portion of a Peloton ride. You may want to do some core classes, crunches, or sit-ups. It will be worth the effort to be able to transfer the effort to your core during a ride (and relieve those legs from doing all the work).

When doing standing portions of a Peloton ride, many riders believe you're in a good position if you can feel the horn of the saddle touch your butt on the downstroke. This means you have correct posture and have positioned yourself correctly. (Many riders also feel that to get the most out of this position, you should also squeeze your glutes whenever you are off the seat.)

There's no question that standing up on your rides can take some adjustment, practice, and possibly new development of your core strength. However, I think you'll agree that becoming oriented to standing rides is well worth the effort and that it opens up one of the most exciting and interesting aspects of Peloton rides.

PELO TIP 53: MOVING THE BIKE TO ANOTHER ROOM

Long after the delivery people are gone and you've gotten to know your bike, you may have a change of heart—or at least a change of aesthetic sense—and decide that the room where you set up the bike might not be its "forever home" after all. Perhaps you have discovered that the Wi-Fi reception in your initial setup room is not ideal and you want to get the bike closer to your router. Unfortunately, if this is the case, you are not going to get the Peloton people to come back; it is up to you (and hopefully at least one other able-bodied person) to make that happen.

You can't easily pick up a 135-pound piece of gym equipment, but it *is* manageable. My advice is to prepare a little bit before you move your bike. Survey the passage from room one to room two. Make sure the surfaces along the way are clear and pick up any area rugs or anything else in the way. With you and your (at least one) helper, pick up the back end and angle the bike forward until it rests on the front conveyor wheels. Then, one of you should move to the front to secure the handlebars—keeping them steady—while the other should continue to hold the back end up. Keeping both hands on the bike, carefully roll the bike to the new room on its front wheels.

When you reach the desired location, carefully lower the bike down into its normal position and make sure it is resting on all four feet. As when you first set it up, it is a good idea to put a mat under the bike and give yourself clearance on both

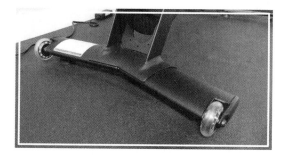

sides to mount and dismount. Be sure to clear space for stretching your arms or working with free weights.

If you find that the bike is rocking after you've moved it, try unscrewing the leveling feet until all four of them are settled on the floor.

PELO TIP 54: FANS

After you spend so much money on the Peloton Bike, it may feel like the least the company could have done was also supply a fan on the handlebars (like many other exercise equipment manufacturers do). However, we've got to play the hand we're dealt. Peloton Bikes don't come with fans, so you'll have to decide if you want to try to correct that.

If you decide you want a fan, you'll find you have many options. At most hardware stores, you can find fans of all sizes. Some will be stand-alone, and others can clip directly to your handlebars.

You're going to get hot as you advance to more strenuous rides. You may find that a well-placed fan really hits the spot!

PELO TIP 55: RIDE LEVELS

Choosing your rides is part of the fun of owning a Peloton Bike. It's also a very subjective thing and will be dependent on your fitness, ability, and personal taste.

If you are not accustomed to spinning—even if you're in good shape and familiar with other exercises—I am still going to suggest you start with the beginner classes. These are the easiest offered and generally low-impact, but they are also perfect for getting used to the bike regardless of your fitness level.

Once you are feeling good about your progress—and don't forget, you can always retake classes if you so desire—I would suggest moving on to some advanced-beginner rides, which, among other things, will introduce you to getting up out of the saddle for short intervals. These classes are longer in duration and will help you build your endurance.

There are also variations within these slightly more advanced classes. For example, there are low-impact rides for all experience levels, which will put less stress on your joints. Peloton instructors also offer Rhythm classes, which can make your workout more like a dance party. They're definitely some of my favorites. Because I love exercising to the rhythm of songs, I sometimes take these even if I can't keep up with some of the drills. I still find them fun, and I think you will, too.

If music is your thing, there are also themed rides set to different genres of music (from Hip Hop to Rock to Country and more). And if you really want to make it a party, try the live DJ classes offered that accompany the instructors and play contemporary songs.

For more structure, try the Metrics rides that "zoom in" and really focus on cadence, resistance, and output. There are also classes that focus on resistance to simulate uphill climbs. And if a laser-focus on cardio is your thing, be sure to take the Heart Rate Zone classes, which'll have you concentrating on the five effort levels, from easy to challenging. The Uber level, in my opinion, is the Power Zone. It is intense but challenging. The graduated organization of all these levels can really help you to achieve your personal fitness goals. The instructor will call out specific zones that have been set up by your personalized output ranges.

Relatively new are the Pro Cyclist class options, which will lead you through a very intense and specialized set of intervals and recovery periods, designed to mimic the training programs used by competitive cyclists.

What about rating your experiences? You might find it annoying (or you might find it satisfying), but every time you complete a ride, you will be asked to rate it. Personally, I would urge you to take the time to rate your rides, because Peloton is really good at taking all the feedback they receive and improving the service. There are also a lot of social media outlets that have their content determined by the company, the instructors, and fans. So try to be constructive and not snarky. If you get engaged and offer real, genuine suggestions, things can only get better. And if you don't tell them what you like or dislike, how will they ever know?

PELO TIP 56: STRIKE THE POSE

When you first tap on your tablet screen, you will find a page that displays all users on your Peloton Bike. Most likely, you will see your own initials and username (the icon), and that is fine for many people. But if you want to add some personality to the board, that's okay, too. A great way to do this is by adding a photo.

To add a photo, first tap on your icon. Then, in the lower left-hand corner, tap your username. On the upper left-hand corner of the page, tap on your icon. Here, on the "Profile Info" page, you will have two choices. You either can take a new photo with the built-in camera on the tablet screen, or you can import an image from Facebook. After you have selected a photo, tap on the save button. And now your profile has a customized photo of you!

PELO TIP 57: SPEAKERS: PROBLEMS AND WORK-AROUNDS

The speakers on the Peloton Tablet are in the back of the device. This can be a problem for some people because when you're using the bike, the speakers are in the rear of the screen, and not pointed directly at the user.

As I've mentioned elsewhere, you can try to adjust the balance between the instructor and the music in an on-demand class by playing around with the volume control, also to be found on the back of the tablet. Alternatively, you can try and raise the volume under settings on the touch screen. However, if this fails to get a good result, you can try plugging headphones into the jack on the right side of the tablet. But cords on many headsets are sometimes not long enough, and you also probably don't want to be wired to the tablet when the exercises get vigorous.

If this is the case for you, it may be time to get wireless earphones—like Apple's AirPods—which work well without the encumbrance of cords or wires.

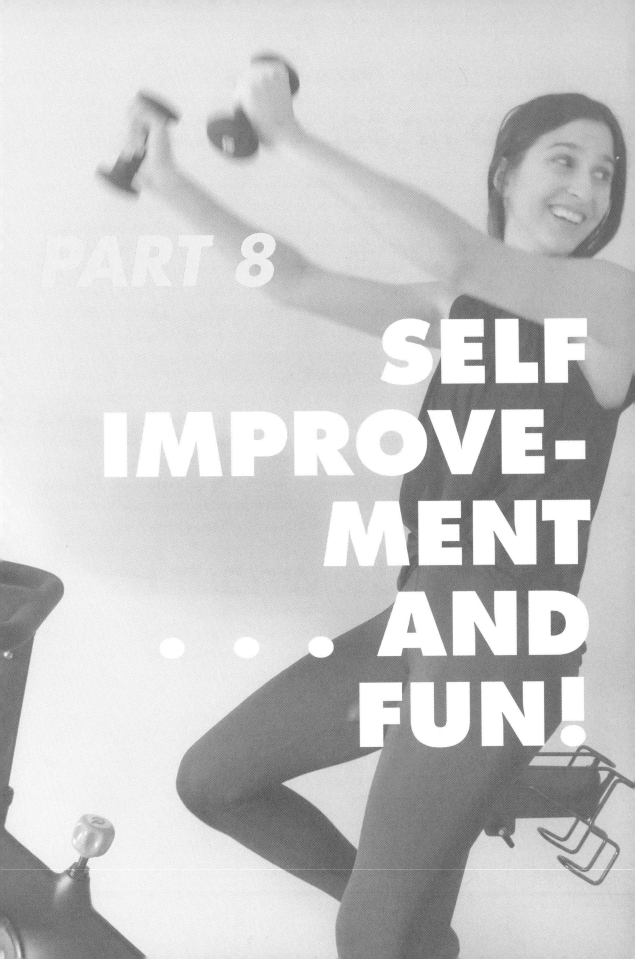

PART 8

SELF IMPROVE- MENT AND FUN!

PELO TIP 58: CALORIES

There are varying schools of thought, which you'll see on social media and elsewhere, suggesting that the calorie counter on the Peloton Bike is not completely accurate. In fact, some Internet wags have been suggesting that each bike is calibrated slightly differently. For a rider like me, that is less of an issue, because I compete with myself on the same bike each time, so what I'm looking for is comparative metrics with other rides that I have done and will do. In other words, for me the question is: Am I burning off more or fewer calories than I did the day before, and what can I try to do tomorrow? Or, put another way, I am not trying to count individual calories so I can know if my latest ride has earned me an extra cookie at dessert. Instead, I am interested in improving on my personal best.

However, there is clearly a big appetite for calorie counting. Many people very much do want to know exactly how many cookies—or fractions of cookies—they may have earned during a workout. And that's okay, too! If you are in this camp, I suggest that you get to know the calorie counter on your Peloton. If you have any doubts about its accuracy—as some users clearly do—a great solution is to simultaneously use another calorie-counting device while on your Peloton, and then compare the results. And, of course, there is always the bathroom scale to really see what is happening!

PELO TIP 59: WEIGHT LOSS

This is definitely not the first book to tell you that the weight-loss journey can be confusing and sometimes frustrating. When you've been working hard on your Peloton, pedaling away like you are in the Tour de France, it can be frustrating to then weigh yourself and realize that you haven't lost a lot of weight . . . or, heaven forbid, find that you actually gained weight. But hey, it happens. Even to Peloton Bike users.

If your only goal is weight loss, I think it's important to remember that while everyone is different, it is generally accepted wisdom that in order to lose weight, you need to exercise *and* eat healthy. Usually doing one without the other is not going to produce the results you want.

But there are other things to keep in mind. Peloton users tend to build muscle as they ride. So riders who begin losing fat, but gaining muscle, don't always see a quick drop-off in their overall weight.

In addition, riding a Peloton tends to improve our endurance, which means we are utilizing the oxygen we take in in a better fashion. That oxygen is moving throughout the body, and this means we are moving better and performing better.

This is just a long way of saying that riding a Peloton will improve your body in a number of healthful ways, but it won't only be weight loss. As for me, I'll take it!

PELO TIP 60: GET CONNECTED

After the state-of-the art quality of the hardware, and the variety and excellence of the instructors offered, the biggest draw for owning a Peloton Bike is probably the sense of community that it builds.

Even though I initially bought my bike because I hated taking in-person classes and exercising in front of other people, I must confess that now, being part of this large group of fellow Peloton users motivates and empowers me—and makes me proud! I find that it definitely stirs up my competitive juices; I sometimes laugh at myself when I see on the Leaderboard that someone who started the ride around the time that I did is now slightly ahead—then I pedal faster or turn the resistance knob, and now I'm in the lead! I have to say, the first time I was really struggling during a ride, and, all of a sudden, someone sent me a virtual "high five," I pushed myself harder just because of that little hand that had popped up on the screen.

Another aspect of being a Peloton rider that can be really gratifying is going on social media sites and reading other riders' stories. The ones that really make me feel connected are those that make me laugh. Those cute dog photos ("Pelo Pups") inspire me or pull at my heartstrings. Once in a while, I'll read posts from people who have lost someone important in their lives, have a sick child, have a husband or wife deployed in a war zone, or used to be sickly or dangerously overweight. They are looking for company, validation, or a spiritual connection. And the responses they get are just beautiful—and the way that becoming a Peloton rider has helped them is remarkable—and they renew my faith in what humans can accomplish.

For me, this is one of the most priceless parts of becoming a rider. I hope that you'll also take advantage of all these possible connections to other riders and the larger ridership community!

PELO TIP 61: IF THE SCREEN TILTS

Your delivery guys should have left you a little tool kit for your Peloton Bike. There are a number of situations in which this kit can come in handy, but perhaps none more useful that dealing with screen tilt.

If the screen on your Peloton should start to tilt over time, take the biggest Allen wrench they provided in your kit and use it to rotate the entire screen left or right. The spot to rotate is located where the arm that holds the tablet attaches to the bike.

Don't worry if your screen begins to rotate; you're not the only rider it has happened to, and the problem is easily fixed with the tools provided!

PELO TIP 62: IS IT ME OR IS IT A UNIVERSAL PROBLEM?

As a Peloton rider, sometimes you're going to experience a problem with your bike, and you may be tempted to assume it is only happening on **your** bike. But is this really the case? Probably, the answer will be no.

Peloton has a way for you to check on all operational systems related to your bike and to verify if your problem is an isolated one.

Go to status.onepeloton.com; there, you can easily see if it is a systems-wide problem. Going to this site will also give you a status from Peloton relating to the problem, such as "Investigating" or "Resolved."

So when and if you do have problems, you'll at least know that you're not the only one!

PELO TIP 63: PELOTON CACHE

Like all the other hardware and software in your technological life, your Peloton tablet has a cache used to store data temporarily, and this is found under your Wi-Fi setting. These caches of data take up storage space and are essentially just junk files. As a rider, you should be aware that if needed, they can be deleted to free up storage space. If you decide to delete them, my personal advice is to call Peloton Support and have somebody walk you through it just to play it safe. Your Peloton Support rep should be happy to help you.

PELO TIP 64: THE PELOTON BRAKE

As much as I am a big believer in total devotion to your exercise routine—without any interruptions whatsoever—emergencies do happen . . . even if it is just the call of nature. Because of this, you're going to want to know about the Peloton brake.

To stop the flywheel from spinning so you can jump off quickly, simply push down on the big orange resistance knob. (Clipping out of your pedal has been dealt with in a different section.) This will allow you to quickly stop the bike and do what you need to do.

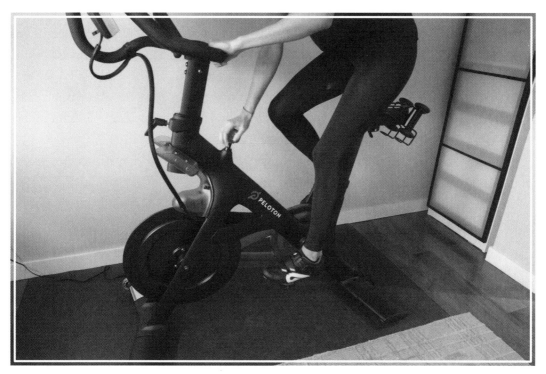

PELO TIP 65: ADJUSTING FOR PAIN

Not to sound like a broken record, but before exercising, you should always consult with a doctor. We are said to live in a "no pain/no gain" world, and for too many of us, therein lies the problem. We push ourselves during our workouts and sometimes ignore serious pain at our own peril. Having said that, there might be things you're doing while riding that are causing the problem. It can be helpful to rule these out to make sure your pain is not caused by something more serious. If you feel any pain or discomfort in your chest, do not assume it is a muscular problem. Go directly to your doctor or the ER.

With that out of the way, there are other types of painful things that can be avoided. As many instructors will tell you, the first thing to do is make sure your butt is positioned on the widest part of the saddle. You'll also want to keep your hips back, your spine and back straight, and your shoulders down away from your ears (no shrugging!).

With regard to your knees, if you are feeling pain in the front of your knee, try raising your saddle and sliding it away from the handlebars. If the pain originates from the back of the knee, do the opposite: lower the saddle and slide the seat toward the handlebars.

If you are experiencing foot or arch pain, the problem may be with your cleats. My suggestion would be to find a local bicycle shop to see if they can help you adjust the cleats.

I cannot say this enough, but there are three other words that are key to minimizing pain when riding: stretch, stretch, and stretch.

And if taking these steps doesn't correct your pain? By all means, check with a medical professional!

PELO TIP 66: CHECK OUT YOUR PROFILE

Many Peloton riders choose not to engage with their apps. While this is, of course, fine to do, I feel it risks the user missing out on a really crucial aspect of the Peloton experience. Keep in mind that with your monthly Peloton subscription, you'll get a lot more than just the ride itself! There are all sorts of activities and metrics contained on the app or available through your tablet.

For the remainder of this book, I want to highlight some of the things you might not know about . . .

When using the Peloton app, I recommend that you check out your "profile" on the lower tool bar. There, you will get a snapshot of your total workouts. By accessing this information, you will immediately see your accomplishments, but, equally important, you will also notice gaps in your routine. Tapping each category (cycling, stretching, meditation, boot camp, cardio, running, strength, walking, yoga), you will be reminded of which instructor you worked out with and be able to see at a glance whether you liked the class or not.

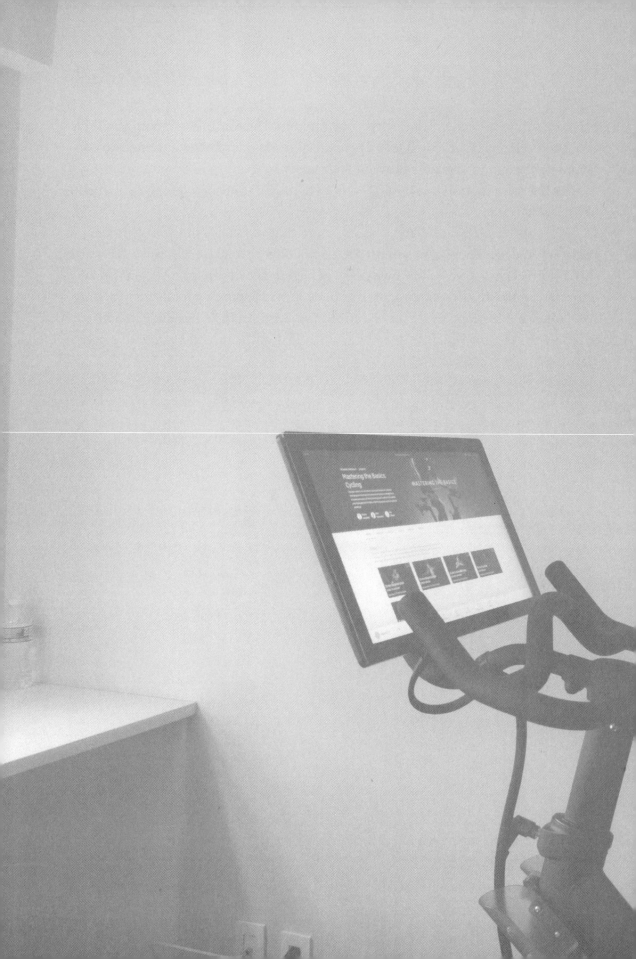

PART 9

CONNECTING TO OTHERS

PELO TIP 67: THE ANNUAL

On the bottom tool bar, you will see a trophy icon and the word "Challenges." You can tap on this word to see some fun little incentives. Relatively new to this section is something called "The Annual." Join this year-long challenge, and the app will track your active minutes on all Peloton platforms. There is a timeline that will show you where you are and keep track of your progress. This should motivate you to keep coming back for more workouts and allow you to check your progress year-over-year.

PELO TIP 68: MONTHLY ACTIVITY CHALLENGE

Another way to increase your desire to return to your bike (or any activity) is by earning "badges." The monthly challenge encourages you to earn a bronze (five days), silver (ten days), or gold (fifteen days) badge for staying active.

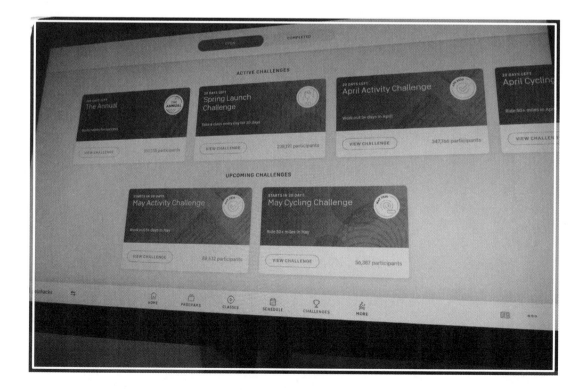

I encourage you to explore the ways in which the monthly activity challenges on your Peloton can become another fun and interesting motivator to your total workout experience.

PELO TIP 69: HOMECOMING

Just like a weekend school reunion, the Peloton Homecoming, formerly known as the Peloton Home Rider Invasion (HRI), is a chance to gather for a couple of days at various locations in New York City for workouts, outdoor community runs, meet and greets with instructors, panels and presentations, concerts, and apparel sales. Peloton negotiates special hotel block pricing for these events. Tickets sell out quickly, and there is always a waitlist. Typically, the tickets go on sale in February for a May weekend celebration.

The event was started in 2016. Over three thousand members from around the country, Canada, Puerto Rico, and the United Kingdom joined the fun. Tickets run around a hundred dollars (and do not include food and lodging).

If you're interested in making an in-person connection with the Peloton community, the Homecoming event may be just the thing for you!

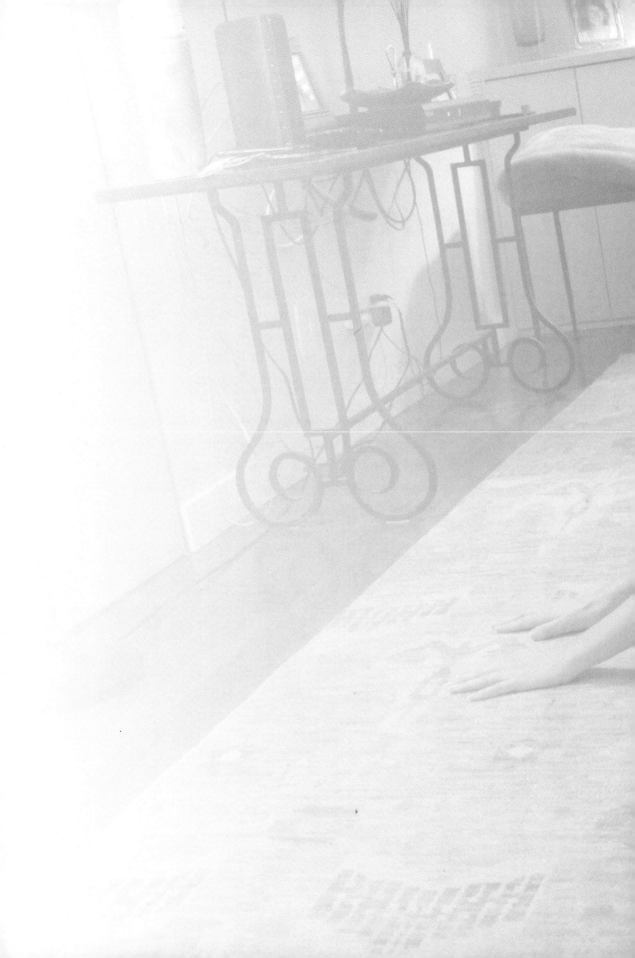

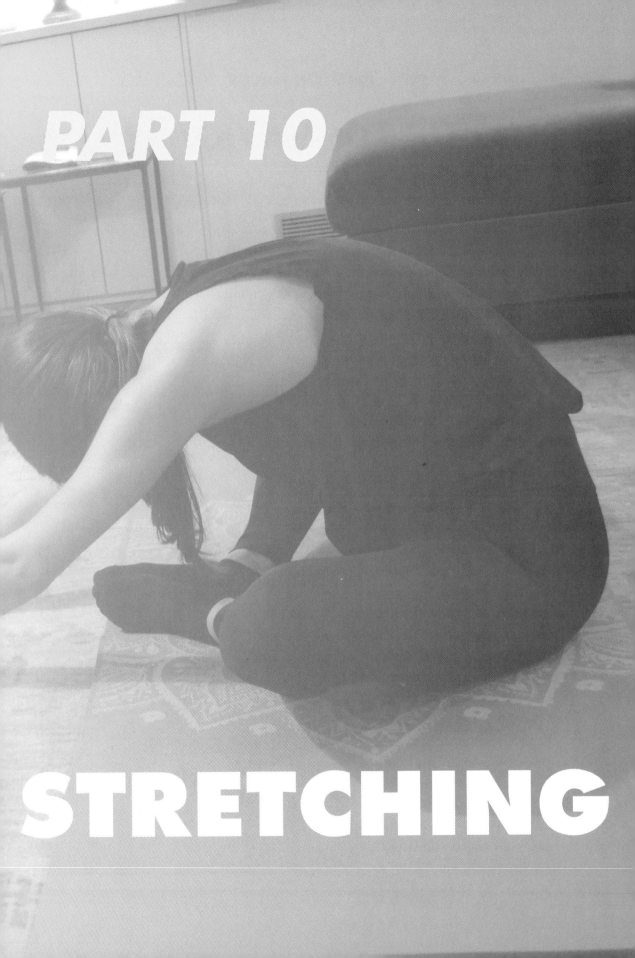

PART 10

STRETCHING

PELO TIP 70: NAVIGATING STRETCHES

I've mentioned the importance of stretching already, and it's nice to see that Peloton also has assets that it provides to help you with stretching.

After tapping "Classes" on the bottom tool bar, you will be taken to a series of tabs representing different types of classes. One of these will be stretching. Tap on "Stretching" to explore it further, and you will immediately notice that Peloton offers numerous stretching exercises ranging from five to fifteen minutes. If you tap on the "Filter" tab, you will see that you have stretching choices that will vary in terms of length, type (e.g., full body, pre- or postride stretch), instructor, music genre, and a miscellaneous tab—called "Sort"—which allows you to choose easiest, hardest, top-rated, most popular, new, or trending. It also gives you the option of choosing "Closed Caption," which I find useful when the music comes up too loud, which can cause me to miss an important direction from the instructor. It is hard to imagine how anyone could be bored with all these choices! (Please note, the tool bar at the top allows you to easily switch between any of the other available Peloton activities.)

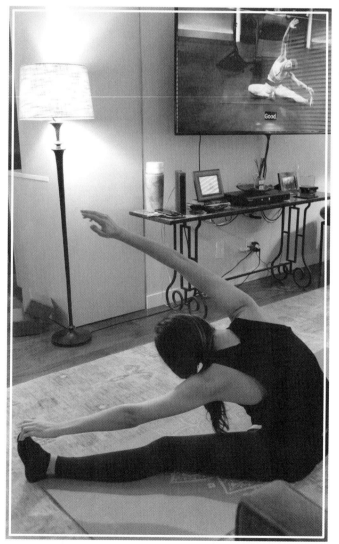

PELO TIP 71: THE FIVE-MINUTE STRETCH

Within Peloton's offerings, you can find many simple exercises that will allow you to stretch your hamstrings, quads, and glutes. A great example that I like is Robin Arzon's five-minute preride warm-up. It's a great way to build up your core and work on your thoracic spine. (It is suggested that you not wear bike shoes during these stretches, so any sneaker or workout shoe will do.) You will do some knee grabs, ankle grabs, calf raises, and static lunges.

After a strenuous ride, you also might like Matt Wilper's five-minute postride stretch, which can help you to restore mobility and accelerate recovery. In just a short period of time, you'll start to loosen up, especially in the calves and hips, which can get really tight when you cycle. (And if you feel that it hasn't gotten you loose enough, you can always take the class again!)

PELO TIP 72: THE TEN-MINUTE STRETCH

Hannah Marie Corbin is one of the instructors I've grown to like most of all. It was a pleasant surprise to learn that not only did she offer a regular ten-minute postride stretch, but that she also offers a Smokey Robinson postride stretch. (And who doesn't love Smokey Robinson?)

Nobody ever said stretching exercises had to be boring. I especially like it when Corbin offers you a little fitness information during a Smokey track!

In this class, you have the option of doing it with shoes or no shoes. A mat and a towel (to put under your knees) are also recommended.

PELO TIP 73: THE FIFTEEN-MINUTE STRETCH

Not everything has to be about the ride! If you have the time—and why not make the time?—I encourage you to try one of the other, longer stretches like Dennis Morton's Full Body Stretch. In this class, you will start off standing and work your way down from the neck, shoulders, and chest—going throughout your body—until you gradually get down on the floor to work on your hips and quads. It is a great exercise class that you could do every day, and all you need is the space as big as your mat.

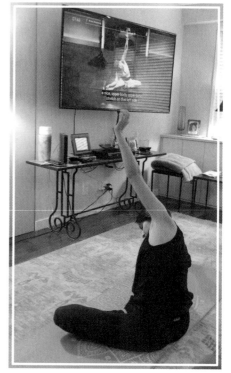

Jess King is another instructor I like very much whom you may want to check out. She shows you each component of a stretch and has your safety and comfort in mind as you proceed throughout the workout. Sometimes the stretches will involve using Styrofoam blocks; if you don't have those, you can use shoeboxes or large books instead!

PELO TIP 74: FOAM ROLLING STRETCHES

A foam roller—just like the Styrofoam blocks—is a minor investment that can become a major asset to your workout and stretching routine. Foam rolling helps to restore mobility, improve blood flow, and can reduce pain, tension, and soreness. The type of foam roller you use is a personal choice—whether it be long or short, hard or soft. Whatever you select, foam rolling exercise is great at relieving the stress in your calves, quads, adductors (the muscles along your inner thighs that stretch from your knees to your groin), hamstrings, hips, chest, and back. You might find the foam roller awkward at first, but the video instruction on the Peloton app is really good and precise and should help you acclimate quickly. If you have to, pause, rewind, and play again. In no time, I expect you will get the hang of it. Your muscles will thank you.

PELO TIP 75: NAVIGATING CYCLING

If you find yourself traveling and can't get on a Peloton Bike, you might desire to simulate the experience that you have at home. Luckily, there are many ways to do this. The best way is probably to bring a tablet or phone in which you have downloaded the Peloton app and get your hands on a traditional exercise bike. (Hopefully, whichever bike you are on will have a tray so you can prop up your device somewhere within eyesight.) Tap on "Classes" on the lower tool bar. Then tap on "Cycling." Then press the "Filter" tab. You will be given a choice of classes lasting from five minutes to ninety minutes. You will see all the levels that you are familiar with, from beginner to Pro Cyclist. You can choose your favorite instructor and music genre and sort from easiest to hardest or by newest, most popular, and top-rated or trending. Of course, you won't be able to see the cadence, resistance, or output metrics that you would be able to access on your Peloton Bike at home. But often you can figure out a way to increase the resistance or speed on the bike at hand. It is not ideal, but at least you have the instructor and great music you are used to at home. If you're doing it like this anyway, you might do the live DJ ride for the fun of it and forget about your metrics!

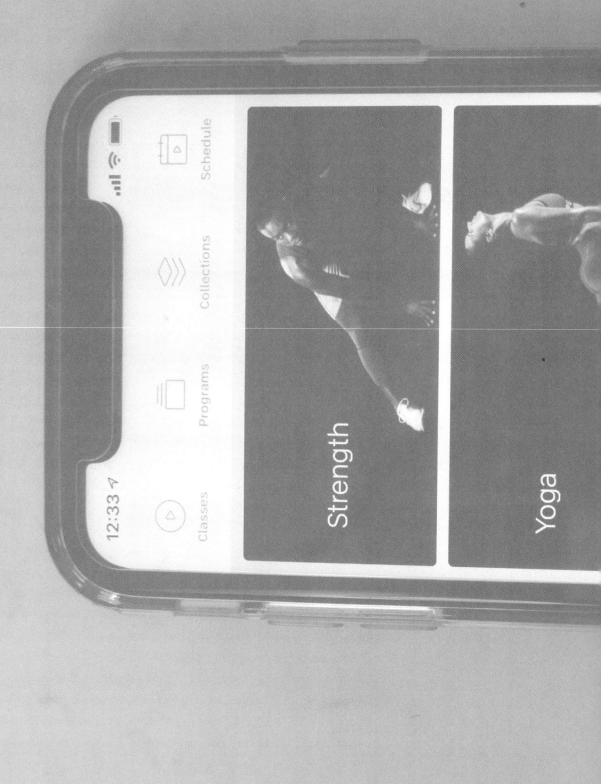

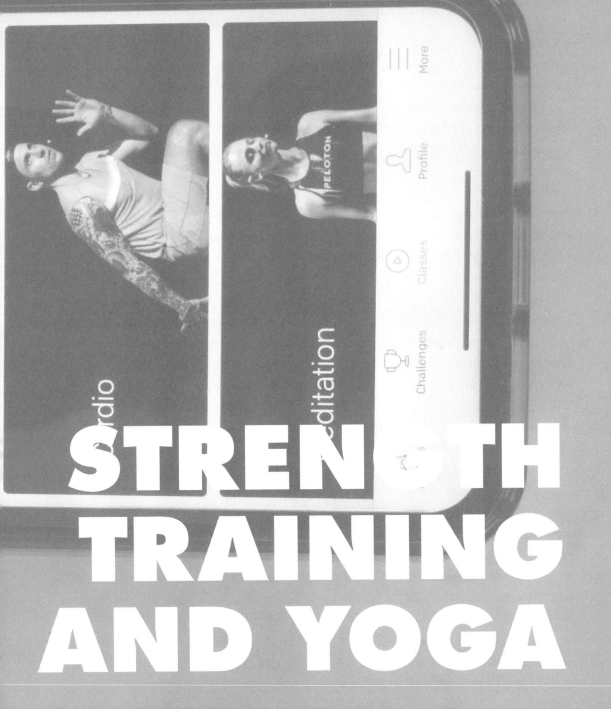

PART 11

STRENGTH TRAINING AND YOGA

PELO TIP 76: NAVIGATING STRENGTH CLASSES

As you progress as a rider, you will almost certainly want to build up your core strength and your endurance. The strength skills classes on the Peloton app are an excellent way to do this.

Let's explore accessing resources that can help you do this. On your home page, start by tapping on "Strength." Then tap on the filter tab, followed by class type. There you will see six choices: lower body, upper body, bodyweight, core, full-body, and strength skills.

The duration of these classes can be as short as five minutes, or as long as thirty minutes. As always, I recommend that you start with an easy five-minute class with one of your favorite instructors. Many of the exercises you'll encounter will already be familiar to you. They will include planks, crunches, obliques, cat cows, bird dogs, forward lunges, squats, and bridges. Some exercises will require dumbbells. (They are recommended at no more than five pounds, but the choice of what to use is ultimately yours.)

I expect you'll have a positive experience with an instructor like Rebecca Kennedy, who believes in an "I do/you do" philosophy. You watch her do an exercise first, and then you follow along. It's easy and fun. Learning the basics and fundamentals will help you derive the optimal effects and avoid hurting yourself.

Even if you already think you know what you are doing, I highly recommend the "Intro to Pushups" class; it will have you doubting what you learned in childhood gym classes and open up a whole new world of getting stronger!

As studies have shown—and as I hope I've already made clear—there are varying opinions with regard to using dumbbells while cycling. My own preference is not to use them. However, this does not mean I can't work on my upper torso when I'm off the bike! Peloton offers some excellent classes that you can do on a mat. Personally, I like the bicep curl exercises. It is a great way to add to your strength routine. I highly recommend that you start with light weights—two-pound dumbbells perhaps—until you build up to heavier ones. Always start on the lower end and work your way up. Your muscles will thank you. The classes will use different tempos and rotations, and, in a very short time, you will start to see an improvement in the shape of your upper arms!

PELO TIP 77: CHOOSING YOUR CLASSES

With thousands of classes to choose from, it can feel difficult to know where to start. The titles of classes are pretty self-explanatory, but there can still be multiple classes with the same name. Using the filters can really help you narrow down the selections to fit your fitness goals and can match your current mood. Do you only have a few minutes, or is it a day in which you have more time to spend on your workout? Have you worked out with the instructor before? What kind of music do you want to listen to? All of this can inform your choices.

Here's one more thing I do before making my final selection: I click on the tab and, before I tap "Start," I look at the rating of the class, the number of ratings it has received, and the level of difficulty. It helps to have these parameters, and they can push you to get over your indecision and have confidence that you're making a good choice!

PELO TIP 78: A CLASS FOR YOUR LOWER BACK

With all this riding and concentration on legs, core, and arm muscles, it can be easy to forget about your lower back. But you neglect this at your own peril. Peloton offers some solid classes to help you avoid injuries to your back. As an example, you might want to take Cody Rigsby's "5 Minute Lower Back," located under the "Strength" tab. All you need is a mat, sneakers, and maybe a towel to protect your body against hard floors. If you feel aspects of the workout are too difficult at first, you can modify until you build up to it. It's a great way to build your strength one step at a time.

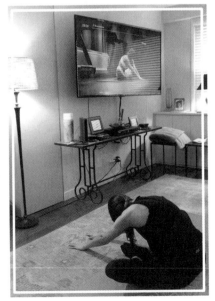

PELO TIP 79: YOGA CLASSES

When people complain to me about the price of an annual subscription to Peloton, I generally only have to ask them what they are paying for gym memberships, personal trainers, and yoga classes—and those conversations usually come to an end! I'm well aware that one loses the immediacy of a live instructor when using the Peloton app, but I'm also very appreciative of the fact that I can replay a difficult position or movement in the comfort of my own home. I can also take the class as often as I wish without any additional charges.

Personally, I'll confess that I approached the yoga classes with some trepidation, and in a way that I hadn't for simple classes in stretching or cycling. For starters, there are those foundational poses that take a lot of practice in order to align, strengthen, and promote flexibility in the body. Add to that the breathing techniques and the meditation aspects that are integrated into the exercise, and I was dubious that the Peloton folks could get me to a place where my body and mind could be trained to become aware of my surroundings and nature and reach a higher consciousness. But I need not have worried!

The first thing I found upon jumping in is that the yoga instructors—like Kristin McGee, Aditi Shah, Ross Rayburn, Colleen Saidman Yee, and Anna Greenberg—were not the usual teachers I encountered in my rides or other exercises. Only Denis

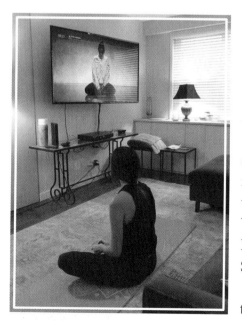

Morton was familiar to me. It was a whole new world, with instructors who were tailored to it. Also, I noticed that Peloton offers the usual five minutes as the basic beginner class but has options that go all the way up to seventy-five minutes.

I would recommend that you start with a five- or ten-minute Basics class for beginners. There are plenty to choose from, and they have names like Cobra, Chair Pose, Tree, Warrior, Half Moon, Locust, Triangle, Upward Facing Dog, Supine Spinal Twist, and Standing Straddle Fold.

As you become more adept, you should try the other class types like Yoga Flow, Restorative

Yoga, Power Yoga, and Yoga Anywhere. For those who are pregnant, there are the Pre- and Postnatal Yoga classes.

On the Peloton Yoga app, you can filter for beginner, intermediate, and advanced, as well as the customary new, trending, popular, top-rated, easiest, and hardest tabs.

As it was for me, I think that your exploration of Peloton's yoga offerings can offer a pleasant surprise!

PELO TIP 80: YOGA AND BREATH

It can be difficult to know where to start when looking at the depth and breadth of the yoga offerings. While there is technically no right or wrong selection, a very good tutorial for the newbie would be something called "5 Minute Basics: Yoga & The Breath." This class, which is highly rated and given a low difficulty score by other users, is taught by Aditi Shah.

In addition to a mat, it is suggested that you have a yoga blanket for this class, and, if you don't have that, you can bring a towel. From the very beginning of this class, you will be thinking of breathing and your movement, inhaling and exhaling.

The ultimate goal of this exercise is to help us reach a balance that allows us to, as Aditi puts it, "relax and calm down, rest and digest."

I can't put it any better than that!

PELO TIP 81: VINYASA-STYLE YOGA CLASSES

A highly rated, but more difficult, class that can help you develop strength and flexibility is Ross Rayburn's "75 Minute Yoga Flow." If you have taken active Vinyasa classes before, then you know what is in store for you. Note that while it is an intermediate class and the length is seventy-five minutes, you are urged not to overdo it and take a break if it gets too intense. In addition to a towel, you are asked to bring Styrofoam blocks. There is a warm-up period that limbers you up before you get to the more intense parts of the class. Things will move more quickly, even the music.

You definitely should work your way up to this one, but I strongly recommend it as a window into this style of yoga.

PELO TIP 82: YOGA AND PREGNANCY

What is especially nice about the yoga exercises for pre- and postpregnancy is that Peloton has designed classes for the different stages of a person's journey to child bearing: first, second, and third trimester, as well as postpregnancy. The exercises are slower-paced and demonstrate modifications more appropriate for those expecting.

It is recommended that you check out the Yoga Basics library if you think these classes might be right for you. In this library, you will find short tutorials on prenatal modification for each trimester. Throughout the catalog, you will be encouraged to do whatever feels comfortable for you: using an extra towel or block to sit on, drinking water, and stopping to rest or use the restroom. The yoga practice here encourages developing strength in your body but also encourages you to rest when you need it. Exercises you do in other classes are greatly modified so you can expand the uterus in a nice way without overstretching things and keep you and the baby safe. The postnatal yoga flow class is designed for those returning to their yoga practice after pregnancy.

It is generally recommended that you wait four to six weeks after giving birth until you get back on the mat. Please always consult your doctor before doing any exercise.

PELO TIP 83: DOUBLE YOUR YOGA FUN

Another intermediate Vinyasa-style yoga class has Ross Rayburn and Kristin McGee teaming up to teach one class. The variety of teaching styles and alternating voices and exercises is a nice touch. If you want a yoga class with more variety, my tip is for you to check this one, "Two for One," out!

PART 12

OTHER WORKOUT OPTIONS

PELO TIP 84: NAVIGATING THE WALKING AND RUNNING APPS

Since you're reading a book about the Peloton Bike, you may be wondering why there's a section on walking and running. But there are a number of ways that walking and running can be enhanced through your Peloton app.

Just as in the other categories within the app, you can filter the classes appropriate for you. Regardless of the type of machine you are on, the basic instruction about your positioning, techniques, and effort will remain the same. The categories you will find on the app: Running Skills, Warm Up/Cool Down, Fun Run, Endurance, Speed, Intervals, and Heart Rate Zones.

I think there are enough classes here to help you hone your skills and make you an efficient runner.

When you're ready to vary your workout and include some running, the Peloton app can be your friend!

PELO TIP 85: NAVIGATING THE GREAT OUTDOORS

Let's say it's a beautiful day and you've just got to get outdoors! Peloton has you covered with a series of audio programs tailored to all sorts of activities you may want to engage in, complete with music and encouragement from some of your favorite instructors. Put on your headphones and take this app out for a spin! Here are just some of the things you might do: "20 minute power walk with Rebecca Kennedy," "45 minute intervals run with Andy Speer," "30 minute Hip Hop fun walk with Jess Sims," "20 minute walk & run with Chase Tucker," "30 minute HIIT run with Matty Maggiacomo," "30 minute Tempo run with Robin Arzon," and a "60 minute Marathon race prep with Matt Wilpers."

Whether you are warming up, walking, going for speed, intervals, or endurance, this feature of your monthly subscription will hopefully motivate and inspire you to take advantage of all the nice weather.

PELO TIP 86: BOOTCAMP

So I tried a program called Bootcamp . . .

I knew I was in for some strenuous exercise just judging by the name of this program on the app, but it was confirmed when I realized that there were no five-, ten-, or fifteen-minute tutorials in this workout. Nope. On this one, you start at twenty minutes and work your way to sixty minutes. The class types here include: Theme, Bodyweight, Low Impact, Body Focus, and Heart Rate Zone. Difficulty levels are beginner, intermediate, and advanced. These exercises are split fifty/fifty between cardio and on the treadmill. And it's all what you might expect!

If you're looking for a bootcamp-type experience from your Peloton workout, the classes so named will give you just what you're looking for. And I speak from firsthand experience!

PELO TIP 87: CARDIO

Looking for a little cardio help? If you go to the "Cardio" tab on the app, you will be introduced to relatively short HIIT classes that may be just what you're looking for. Alex Toussaint's "5 Minute Cardio" will have you doing all sorts of intense exercises like jumping jacks, triceps dips, running in place, and push-ups. His instructions are clear, and he telegraphs what you will be doing next. The idea is to go hard and get your day started in an energetic and efficient way. Phew!

PELO TIP 88: MEDITATION

Back at the beginning of this book, I shared how my wife and I, fed up with feeling out of shape and overweight, decided to invest in this expensive piece of exercise equipment and committed ourselves to the monthly subscription plan. It was a gamble and a risk, of course, just like all the gyms we had joined through the years and then abandoned. Two things had always gotten in my way when it came to exercise (besides simple laziness): boredom and the sheer inconvenience of getting to the health club on an inclement day or when other appointments made it impractical to go someplace to work out, get back home, shower, and go back out again. Who knew that the Peloton classes would overcome the first problem and this beautiful bike in the room next to my bedroom would solve the second!

But what I had not anticipated was how much we would embrace the Peloton holistic approach to wellness. Getting a good spinning workout was what we thought about when we made the purchase. But little did we realize that there were all these other benefits that came with the app. Stretching, yoga, strength training . . . these were all value-adds.

This leads me to the last program category: meditation. Resting the mind and attaining a state of consciousness are things that have eluded me for most of my life. From childhood on, there was no stillness or bliss for me. And letting go was not something I did very well.

On a recent trip to Japan, my wife and I learned about the Japanese monk, Dosho, who discovered Zen on a visit to China. And through the years, I had also learned about how meditation had originated in India several thousand years ago, and, of course, I knew about Transcendental Meditation as practiced in America. But I just couldn't find a way into it . . . until now.

Not to get too spiritual on you, but I once found myself doing a five-minute Basics class—"My First Meditation with Aditi Shah"—and had a special experience. The class was a short primer to the practice, and I did a breath-based meditation. Of course, it was too short to have a significant impact on my life, but it was still a small spark of something great.

Rather than get on with my day right then and there, I went back into the app, and, using the filter, I found that Aditi had many other meditation classes, and so I tried some of those. I had a positive response to these, as well. Over time, I felt myself "giving in" to the spirit of the classes. They were soothing. I soon felt like a walking cliché, but there was a real and new mindfulness that I was able to experience. I even tried her guided meditation to help me fall asleep at night, and while it has not yet solved all my insomniac tendencies, it may have helped a bit.

I have tried other instructors in meditation available through Peloton, and they have helped me, as well. And just as in the Outdoor programs, there are audio classes that you can listen to when you are away from home and wish to engage in meditation. In particular, I like to listen to Kristin McGhee when I commute. On the days I have listened to her, I have not checked on texts or emails while taking part in this meditation exercise—and that's saying something! It is a great way to start the day.

CONCLUSION

Like riding the bike and taking the classes, writing this book has been a lot of fun. (Not so much the writing itself perhaps, but the chance to get to know a piece of equipment and the attendant software that comes with it that has already given me such pleasure.)

I knew with the first keystroke that so much of what I was going to present here was going to be very subjective. How could it not be? Everyone who picks up this book will be at a different fitness level and will have different experiences with technology. It is hard to be "everyman" to all readers.

This book is unofficial. Peloton did not ask me to write it. Perhaps they will find fault with parts of it. Perhaps you will. That's okay! All errors are mine. With all the nonfiction books I have ever read, it has been my belief that if I could learn a few things I didn't know, then it will have been worth the read. That is my fervent hope in writing this. I didn't set out to get rich or win any literary prizes. My sole reason for writing it has been that I believe there are people like me out there who will really benefit—and perhaps benefit tremendously—from giving a Peloton Bike a chance.

Now, through the reading of these tips, maybe you know things about Peloton Bikes that you didn't know before. If this is what I've accomplished, then I'll be more than happy!

I sincerely believe that a Peloton Bike is one of the most important fitness innovations to arise in modern history. It takes advantage of almost every contemporary technological innovation and uses them to allow riders to create custom fitness programs that can be engaged virtually anywhere—and at any time—with a level of immersion also set by the user. If you are interested in getting fit, but perhaps have been waiting until the stars aligned to make it possible, I think this is your sign that the stars are finally configured just right! I hope you will look seriously at the Peloton Bike, and my earnest wish is that you get as much out of it as I have.

And to all my fellow riders out there, see you on the Leaderboard.

ABOUT THE AUTHOR

MARK A. GOMPERTZ has been a publisher of many *New York Times* bestselling books for over four decades. He has edited several books on fitness and health. A life-long couch potato, Gompertz is now an active and proud Peloton owner.

ACKNOWLEDGMENTS

After so many years of publishing other people's books, I finally got a taste of my own medicine. Like the proverbial case of doctors who make poor patients, I can't imagine how many eye rolls I received from my talented collaborators on this project. Speaking of doctors, I want to thank Scott Kenemore, whose book doctoring kept me honest. My editor extraordinaire, Caroline Russomanno, lived up to the reputation other authors have written about through the years. Kirsten Dalley deserves a tremendous round of applause for her production expertise. For his beautiful cover, I am grateful to Brian Peterson. Thanks to my life long friend, Kevin Goldman, who knows more about media than anyone on this planet. Helping get the book out in the world and noticed, I thank Skyhorse Publicity Director, Kathleen Schmidt. Of course, I would be remiss if I didn't express my gratitude to the entire Skyhorse staff (the little engine that could). For his tremendous encouragement and support, I want to thank my publisher, Tony Lyons.

I'm extremely appreciative to Daniel Spielsinger and Allie Weber for modeling for the photos. I can't imagine what a disaster this book would have been if we had gone with the original plan of me posing. A special shout-out to Eric Spielsinger, whose computer knowledge prevented me from losing the manuscript somewhere in the ether. To my sons, Zachary and Julian Gompertz, I thank them for inspiring me always. To my photographer and better half, Penny Lowy, no words can express my love and adoration.

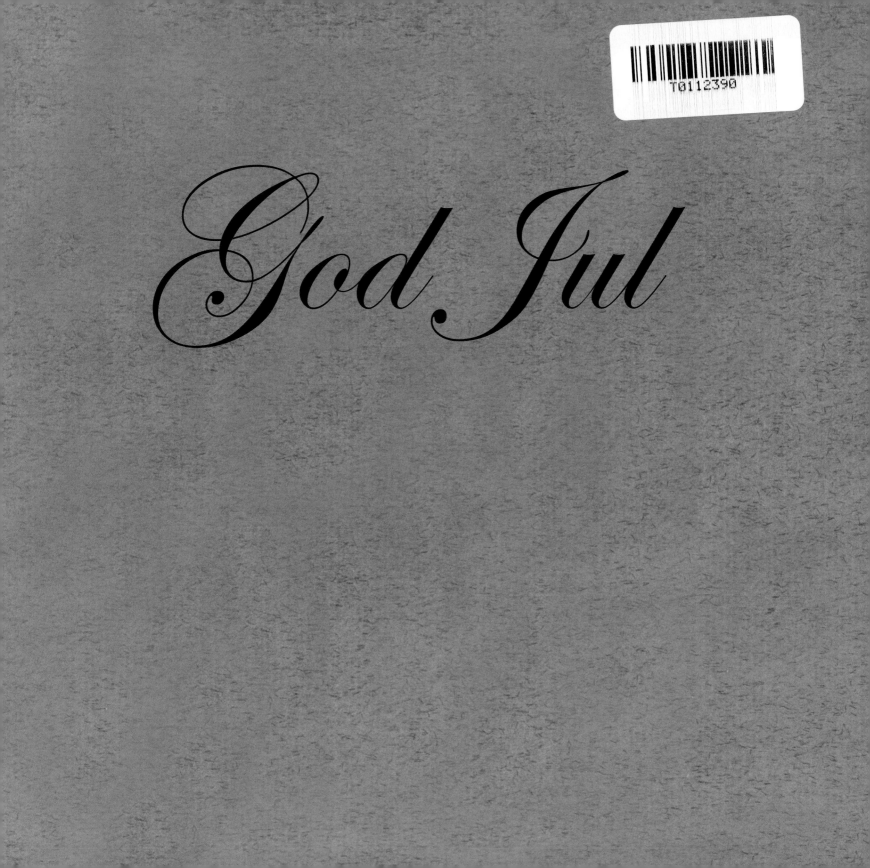

God Jul

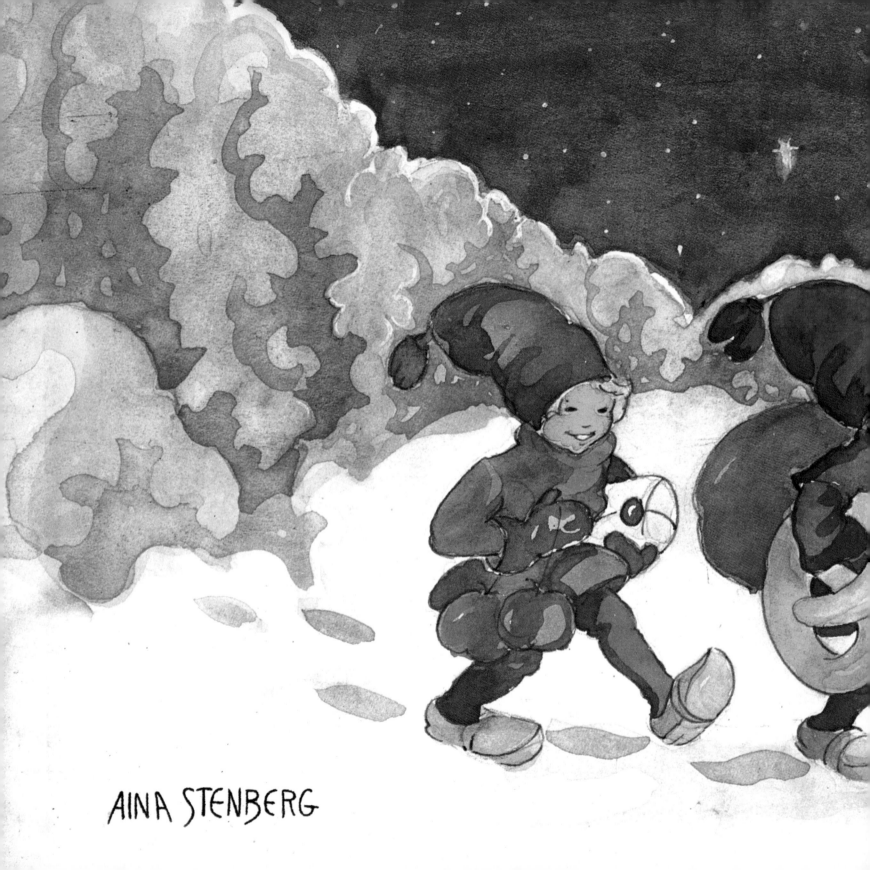

AINA STENBERG

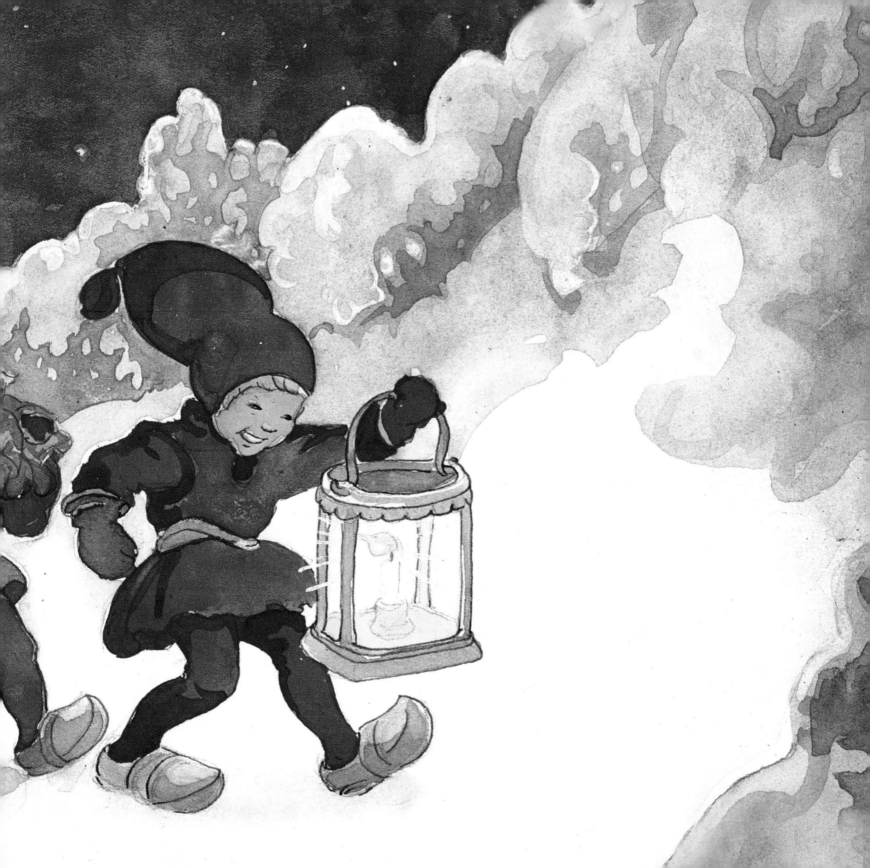

BREFKORT.

(ADRESSEN ANBRINGAS Å DENNA SIDA.)

Sverige 35

Till Anna-Lisa Cederlund,
Karin Jansson MasOlle och
Torsten Pehrsson med
tack för ovärderlig hjälp.

To Anna-Lisa Cederlund, Karin Jansson MasOlle, and Torsten Pehrsson with thanks for invaluable help.

Copyright © 2009, 2021 by Anders Neumuller

www.skyhorsepublishing.com

10 9 8 7 6 5 4 3 2 1

Library of Congress Cataloging-in-Publication Data is available on file.

Paperback ISBN: 978-1-5107-6831-4
Hardcover ISBN: 978-1-60239-755-2
eBook ISBN: 978-1-62873-253-5

Printed in China

Previous pages: Aina Stenberg, Eskil Holm, Stockholm 1940 (reprinted 1978).

Cover: Jenny Nyström, Axel Eliassons Konstförlag, Stockholm 1908.

Design: Anders Neumuller
First published by Bonnier Fakta 1978

The reproduction rights for the Jenny Nyström and Curt Nyström Stoopendaal-motifs in the book were obtained from Axel Eliasson AB Konstförlag, and the Aina Stenberg motifs from Karin Jansson and Britta Yngström.

Anders Neumuller

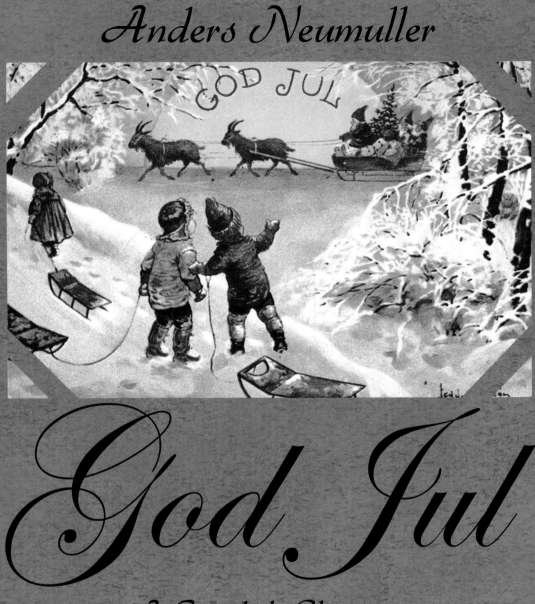

God Jul

A Swedish Christmas

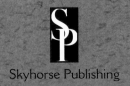

Skyhorse Publishing

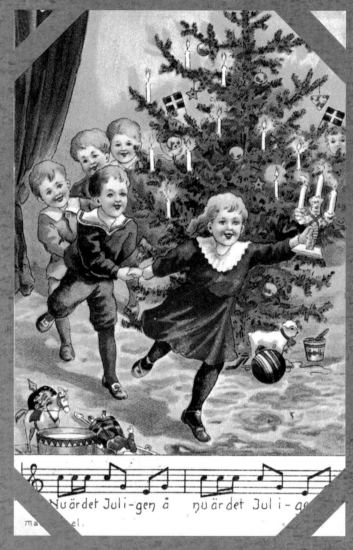

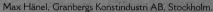

Max Hänel, Granbergs Konstindustri AB, Stockholm.

Contents

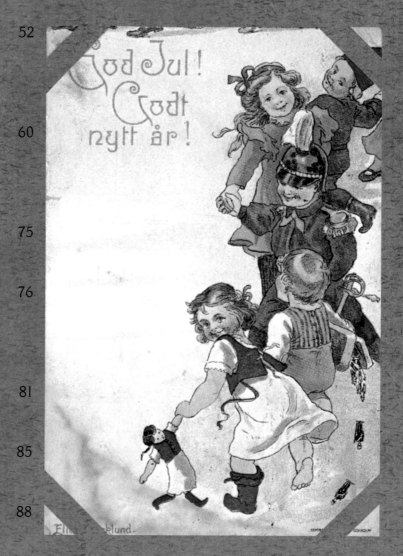

92   Ellen Björklund, Centraltyckeriet, Stockholm 1907.
The card was an insert in the Midwinter Christmas
magazine that was published by Frölén & Comp., Stockholm.

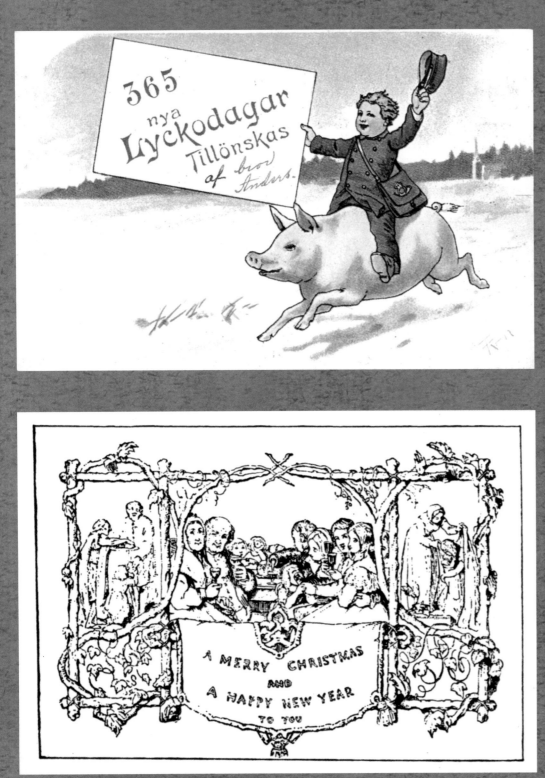

When You Are Waiting for Something Good...

The Celebration of the Year   It is no coincidence that in Sweden the most important celebration of the year takes place during the darkest and most inhospitable season of the year. Christmas brightens Swedish life and gives us something to look forward to during the rest of the year. Christmas traditions have changed almost entirely during the last four to five generations. Many of what are considered to be ancient traditions, handed down from generation to generation, were actually unknown to Swedish forefathers. We have let go of customs that have lost their significance and acquired new and imported ones that we feel have added something more meaningful to the celebration of the year.

The Visual Christmas Ideal   One of Sweden's youngest traditions is the Christmas card. It would be hard to imagine Christmas without them. When Swedes conjure up a picture of Christmas in their imagination, they see something that has been depicted on a Christmas card. The background and the people may be a bit different, but the set-up has been available for sale on a 4 × 6-inch piece of cardboard. Swedish image of a real Swedish Christmas has been shaped by decades of holiday cards. This is where the Christmas goat, the Christmas buffet, the Christmas pig, Santa, the Christmas tree, the early morning church service—yes, even the Christmas spirit first appeared in a picture format and gradually became Swedish visual ideal of Christmas. The Christmas celebration is a romantic quest for more secure times of the past. This nostalgic quest is also one of the reasons why we see so few entirely modern Christmas cards. Publishers try to introduce more international motifs and contemporary artists, but most people still choose older, beloved motifs from Christmases past.

Facing page:

TR-n (Torvald Rasmussen),
Le Moine & Malmeström
Konstförlag, Göteborg 1904.

J.C. Horsley, R.A., Joseph
Cundall of New Bond Street,
London 1846 (1881).

Anonymous German card with
glitter, 1892.

AF (Alfred Schmidt), 1895.

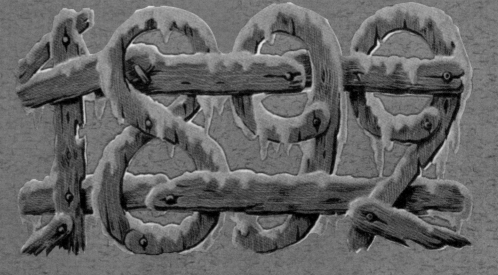

The First Christmas Card   How did the Christmas card come about? There are many theories. Greeting cards in some form or another have actually been used throughout the ages. At the time of the birth of Christ, the Romans sent palm leaves or small gifts to each other as a symbol of victory and success. In Japan there is a very old tradition of giving Surimono cards to friends and relatives on the Japanese new year. (The explorer Sven Hedin had a Chinese New Year's greeting card from 300 A.D. in his collection.) The oldest European new year's greeting still in existence dates back to the 14th century. Toward the end of the 18th century names day cards became popular in Germany. Each calendar day was dedicated to a saint and, on the day, you would send greeting cards to any acquaintances who had the same name as the saint. This was much easier than trying to remember birthdays. Half a century later, the first new year's card appeared in England and it was not many years after this that Henry Cole ordered the very first Christmas card in 1843. Sir Henry—his title derived not from the invention of the Christmas card, but for his founding of the Victoria and Albert Museum—had started a phenomenon. The artist John Calcott Horsley depicted the yuletide message with a happy family seated around an extravagant Christmas meal. Three generations—children, parents, and grandchildren—raise their glasses in a toast to a merry Christmas and a happy New Year. The temperance lobby of the time protested against the motif and were not appeased by the vine-framed side panels showing the less fortunate being fed and clothed. The card was printed in 1,000 copies that were individually hand-colored by the artist. Just two Christmases later, the Royal Mail distributed 25,000 Christmas cards.

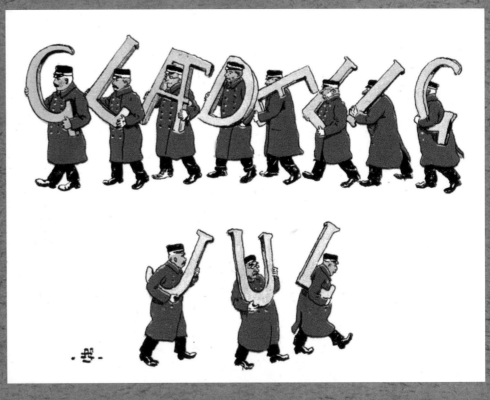

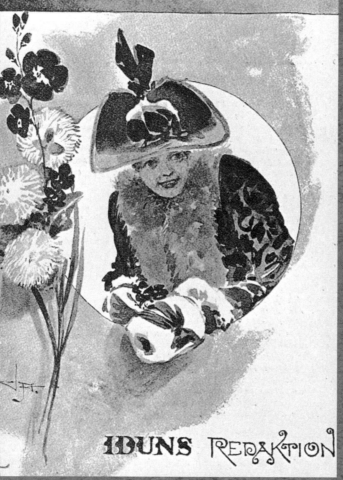

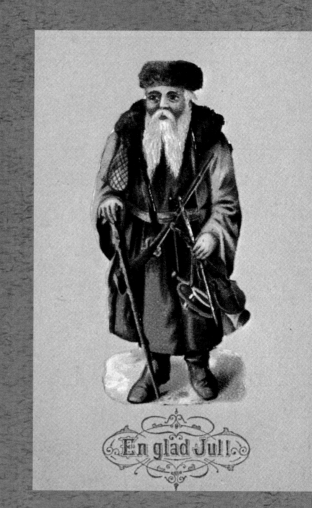

The Golden Age of the Christmas Card   Starting off as a rather exclusive phenomenon, the Christmas card got its big breakthrough in the 1760–70s when people in large parts of Europe started sending them to each other. One reason for the spread of this custom was that the price of the cards and the postage came down considerably. At the same time, introduction of oil printing meant that the chrome lithographic method replaced hand-coloring. The foremost artists of the time were engaged and competitions with large cash awards were announced to bring in new motifs. In England alone, as many as a quarter of a million different motifs were produced as Christmas cards before the turn of the century.

Tulle and Silk Ribbons   The very first Christmas cards were sent or given to the recipients in envelopes just like normal letters. The envelope made it possible for the card to be decorated with pressed flowers, tulle, velvet cut-outs, cloth appliqués, silk fringes, and reliefs in gold. Snow and ice was depicted with glitter made of glass or metal, cotton wool, and tin foil. The card would sometimes incorporate a mechanism that changed the picture, or three-dimensional components that could be folded out. Realistic imitations of cigarette butts, false teeth, bacon, corkscrews, hairpins, and coins were popular. What connection these had to Christmas was anybody's guess.

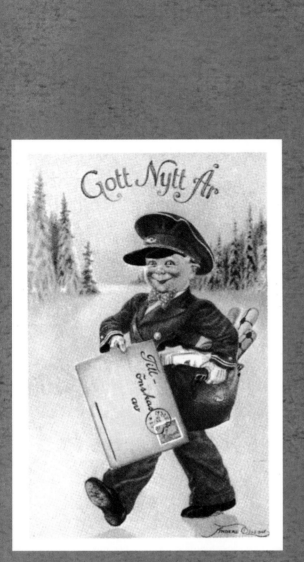

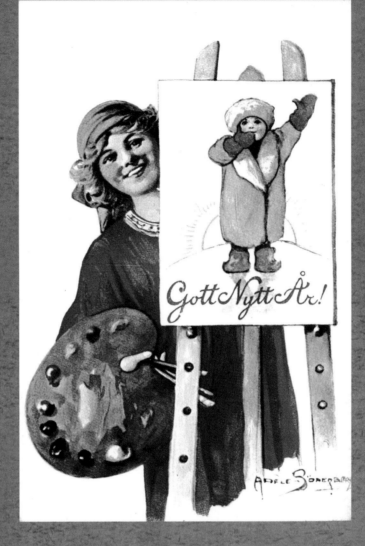

Swedish Christmas Cards   When the postcard was introduced toward the end of the 19th century, the postal service had to bring in extra staff to handle the flood of Christmas cards. Competition between publishers increased and the artistic quality declined. The least expensive production was in Germany, and subsequently large parts of Europe were consuming German angels, Santas, and rather monotonous winter landscapes. It took a long time for Swedish Christmas card publishers to free themselves from the German dominance. The Danes were somewhat more successful, and for this reason there are many old Swedish Christmas cards that read *Glaedelig Jul* instead of *God Jul*. The essentially Swedish Christmas cards only started appearing after the turn of the last century. They became so successful that Swedish motifs were sold in Scandinavia, Russia, Estonia, Latvia, Lithuania, and in the Swedish settlements of North America.

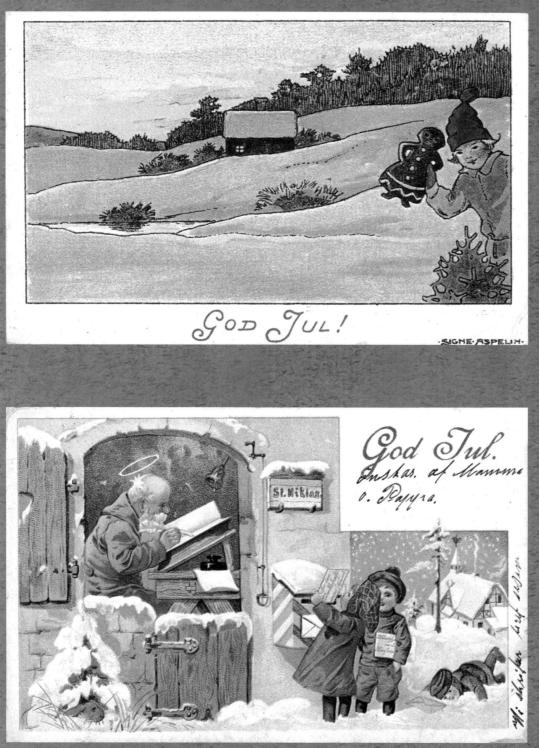

Signe Aspelin, Axel Eliassons
Konstförlag, Stockholm after 1910.

German Christmas card imported
by Åhlén & Holms Konstförlag,
Insjön 1905.

GOD JUL!

·SIGNE·ASPELIN·

God Jul.

St. Niklas

Christmas, a Harvest Festival The winter season is taxing. In the countryside, the progressively shorter days had to be filled with more and more work. The climatic conditions in the Nordic countries meant that a good harvest could never be taken for granted, and therefore there was no celebration until the threshing was done. And that was around Christmas time. For Swedish forefathers, this was the end of a long and hard year of work, without any vacation. At last, all the stores were filled and it was time to enjoy the fruit of their labor. This was the Christmas of the agrarian society and of past times. In Sweden there have never been special harvest celebrations of the kind they have in southern Europe in the fall, so a Swedish Christmas is essentially an old harvest festival.

The Timing "And it came to pass in those days, that there went out a decree from Caesar Augustus that all the world should be taxed." These are the first lines of the story of Christmas (Luke 2:1). But the events that are retold did not actually take place at the time of year that we celebrate it today. Celebrating the birth of Christ in December has a pagan background. We do not know exactly when Jesus Christ was born, but historically the day has been defined as January 6. When Christianity was introduced in the Nordic countries, the newly selected time for Christ's birth coincided with the pagan Midwinter sacrificial feast. From the Midwinter feast, we have only retained the copious eating and drinking and the word *Jul*. *Jul* has probably also existed in other Germanic languages but has been Christianized to Christmas (Christian mass) and *Weihnacht* (the holy night).

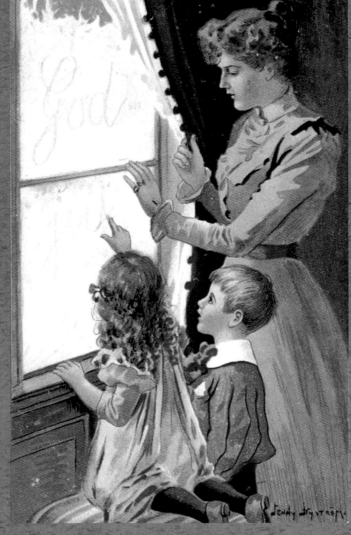

Anders Olsson,
Bacco 1965.

Jenny Nyström, Axel
Eliassons Konstförlag,
Stockholm 1905.

The Waiting Game   The time leading up to Christmas
has always felt extra long for children. Countless are the
wish lists that were written during this time. To help them
count the number of days left until Christmas, children
are given advent calendars. The first such calendar was
published in 1934 by the League of Swedish Female Scouts
and designed by the famous Christmas card artist Aina
Stenberg MasOlle who continued to do the design for the
next thirty years. Eventually, Walt Disney and Swedish
television started producing other popular versions of the
calendar. Ten years before the advent calendar, the advent
candlestick was introduced to enable adults to count the
days left until Christmas.

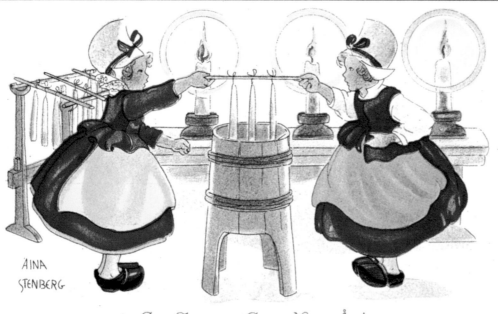

GOD JUL OCH GOTT NYTT ÅR!

Busy Times

Christmas Preparations The first preparations for Christmas used to start during the summer. That is when the curdling of the Christmas cheese was done, and toward the late summer, nuts were collected for all the sweets. Apart from this, most of the main tasks were saved until November. Animals were to be slaughtered, *lutfisk* prepared, and Christmas beer brewed. At the same time the farmer had to get in and thrash the harvest, dig up the potatoes, and pick the last of the vegetables. The fields had to be prepared for the spring sowing and all the tools checked and stored away. Then there was all the firewood that would be needed for the long winter ahead—just one of the myriad tasks that needed to be completed. You have to wonder what we have to complain about these days.

Useful Gifts Swedish forefathers seemingly had an informal open-house format for their celebrations. The more formalized generosity probably came with the Christian influence. Households always had to have gifts in preparation for visitors as no one was to leave the house empty-handed. During a time when the economy was based on subsistence production, bread was the most common gift, but food items, aquavit, fabric, and candles were good substitutes. Tenement soldiers, pastors, parish clerks and any employees were also paid in kind, while the parish poor were given a taste of the bread.

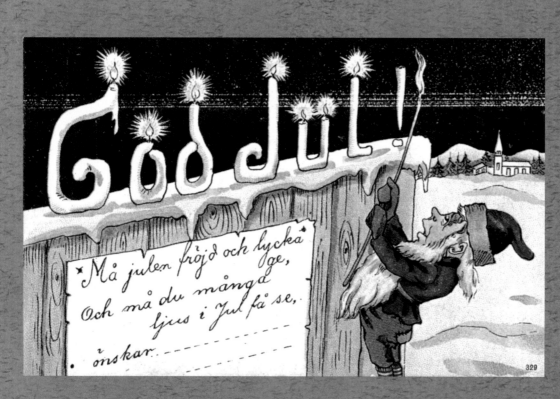

God Jul!

Må julen fröjd och lycka ge,
Och må du många ljus i Jul få se,
önskar.

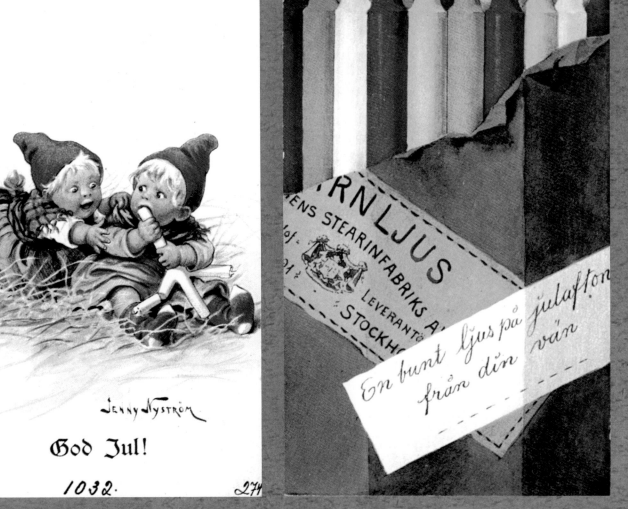

Jenny Nyström

God Jul!

1032.   274

Previous page:

Aina Stenberg, Eskil Holm,
Stockholm 1946.
Anonymous 1905–1910.

Jenny Nyström, Axel
Eliassons Konstförlag,
Stockholm 1909.

Anonymous, Le Moine &
Malmeström Konstförlag,
Göteborg 1910.

Lit Candles Lit candles have become one of the most important ingredients of the Christmas celebration. This came about only after electric light became commonplace. Prior to this, candles were an everyday necessity, and candle-making was part of the normal Christmas preparations. Candles with branches were used to spread light on the Christmas table. Candles with three branches were christened "Trinity Candles." Originally, each family member was designated one branch of the candle and how long and bright each branch burnt became one more way to foretell the future. Above all, the burning of the branches predicted whether it would be the master of the household or the mistress who would die first.

After the electric light had lost its novelty value, it was largely precluded from the Christmas celebration. Churches that used electrical lighting (even with electronic flickering) during the rest of the year, turned it off during the Christmas holidays. Today with a greater awareness of the hazards of fire, electric lights are the norm on Christmas trees as well as on window decorations.

15

Anders Olsson, Sago
Konst AB 1930.

Lisa Lindberg, Granbergs
1891–1905 (with
Swedish-Norwegian
union flag).

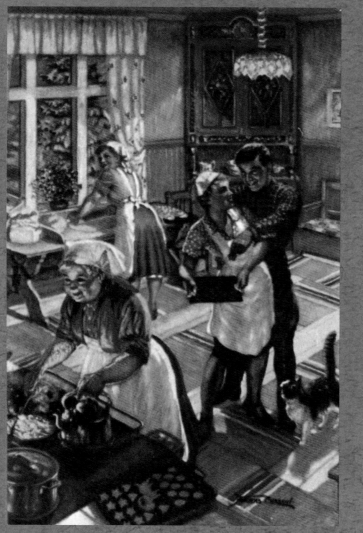

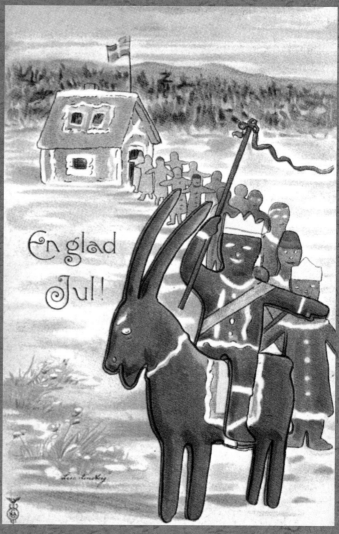

Christmas Baking   About a week before Christmas, it was time to start baking. First in line were the gingerbread cookies as they did not need to be fresh. Called *pepparkakor* (pepper cookies) in Sweden, they used to be baked with real pepper and not specifically for Christmas. Saffron buns, which today are a Christmas specialty, were also eaten year-round. Special for Christmas at that time were the shapes given to the saffron buns and the gingerbread cookies which were also used as Christmas tree ornaments and decorations. Apart from shapes like roosters, pigs, horses, hearts, stars, men, and women, the gingerbread dough was also used to make entire landscapes, with houses, churches, and carriages that were kept until the Christmas tree was stripped and thrown out at the end of the holidays with a party. The pig, by illustrator Einar Nerman, and the other decorative animals were originally symbols of fertility, appearing as growth demons.

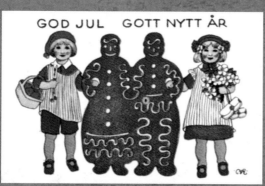

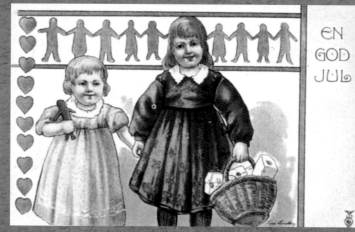

B.E. (Britta Elfström)

Lisa Lindbergs,
Granbergs
1891–1905.

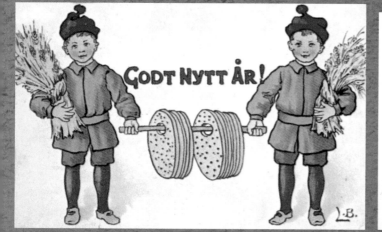

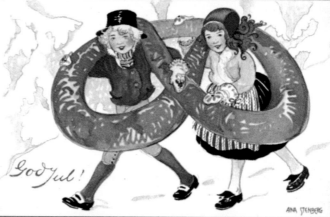

L.B., Eskil Holm,
Stockholm.

Aina Stenberg,
Eskil Holm, Stockholm.

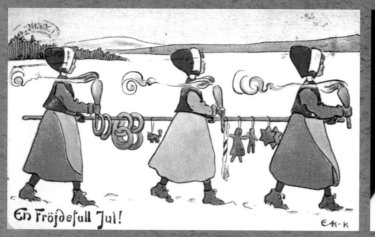

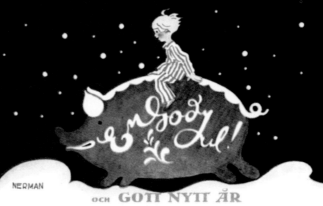

E.K-K., Paul Heckscher
1920.

Einar Nerman,
Nordisk Konst.

17

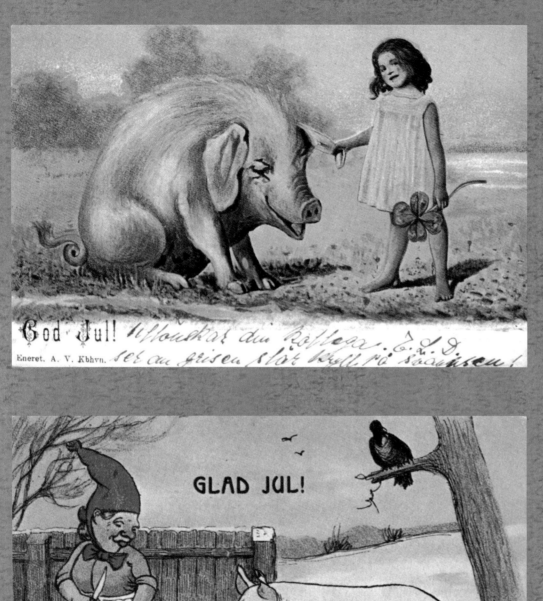

God Jul!

Eneret. A. V. Kbhvn.

GLAD JUL!

Eneret, A.V., Köpenhamn
1891–1905.

Anonymous 1905–1910.

Slaughter   On Anna's Day, December 9, it was time to soak the lutfisk. This was also the first time the Christmas beer could be tasted. The slaughter had already begun, especially for sheep and cattle which would only get progressively thinner as the winter season set in with a vengeance. For the pigs, the situation was the opposite: It was better to slaughter them as close to Christmas as possible to allow them to get fatter. The cheerful, fat pigs on many a New Year's card were somewhat of an anomaly but also indicative of the pig having become a Christmas symbol with a value beyond the Christmas table.

Piggy   The main figure of Christmas is definitely Santa, but the pig is a strong runner-up. The Christmas goat ranks third, at best, in the Christmas hierarchy among mythological figures, all of which were outdistanced by children, especially on Christmas and New Year's cards. The pig is often depicted as Santa's friend and close associate. The more human-looking the pig, the closer is his relationship with Santa and humans. Indeed, in the olden days the gingerbread man and gingerbread woman were called Nisse and Nasse, respectively. Nisse is the Swedish word for the legendary good-natured elf, while Nasse is the nickname for a pig. On one of her cards, Jenny Nyström even painted a *Nisse & Nasse AB* on a truck indicating a pig helping Santa transport Christmas gifts. That pig had definitely risen through the ranks! Today, Nasse has merged with Nisse into Santa's helper.

Jenny Nyström, Axel Eliassons Konstförlag, Stockholm 1906.

Anonymous embossed Danish card from 1911.

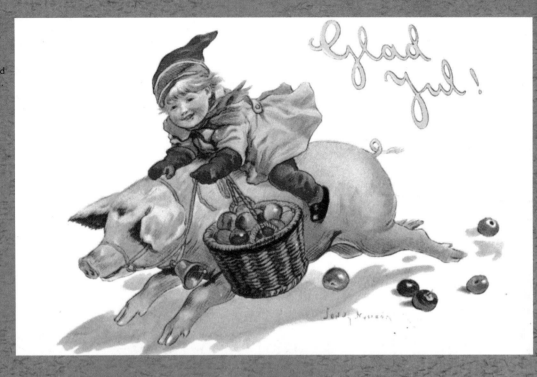

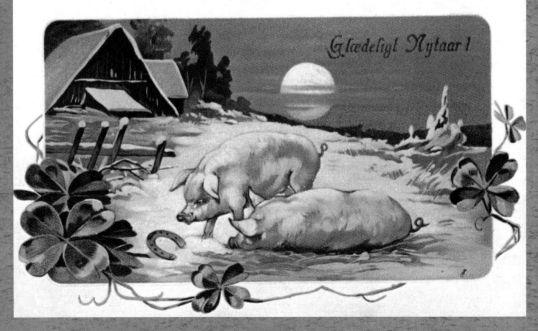

Christmas Card Motifs   "Flowers, Santas, everything possible and impossible from the whole world, from all seasons have been forced to become part of the Christmas card," laments Gleeson White in his book, *Christmas Cards and Their Chief Designers* (1895). He plowed through some huge Christmas card collections. The largest British collection encompassed 163,000 Christmas cards in 700 albums weighing over 6 tons.

As time went by, Christmas card producers had a better idea of what sold, and the huge variety in motifs diminished. Since almost all Christmas cards undergo aesthetic consideration before they are sent, they are a very good reflection of people and the culture they live in. Hence, the Christmas pig's evolution from the ham to family happiness has a significant symbolism.

Christmas Card Psychology   In Great Britain, the Christmas card phenomenon was given serious consideration, and British psychoanalysts even claimed to be able to read the character of a person by his or her choice of cards. The results published in 1963 are not that sensational: "Large Christmas cards are sent by people who have an inferiority complex or are afflicted with some type of exhibitionism."

19

Jenny Nyström,
Axel Eliassons
Konstförlag,
Stockholm 1911.

Anonymous
German card.

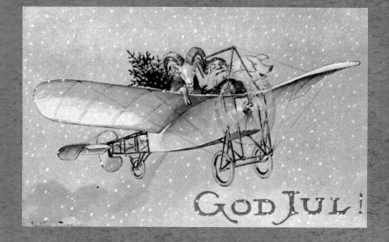

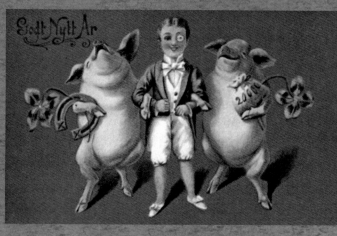

Jenny Nyström,
Axel Eliassons
Konstförlag,
Stockholm 1902.

Jenny Nyström, Axel
Eliassons Konstförlag,
Stockholm 1902.

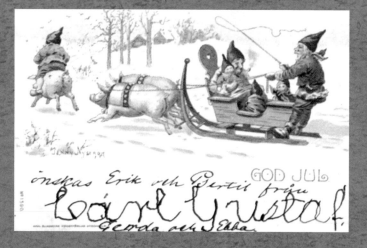

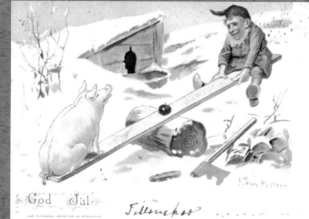

Anonymous, C.N:s
LLj., Stockholm 1946.

Jenny Nyström, Axel
Eliassons Konstförlag,
Stockholm 1908.

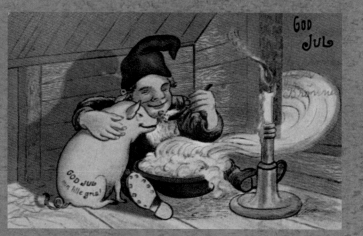

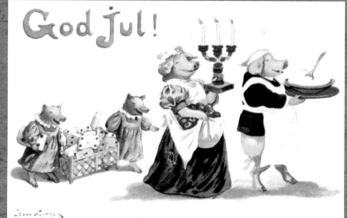

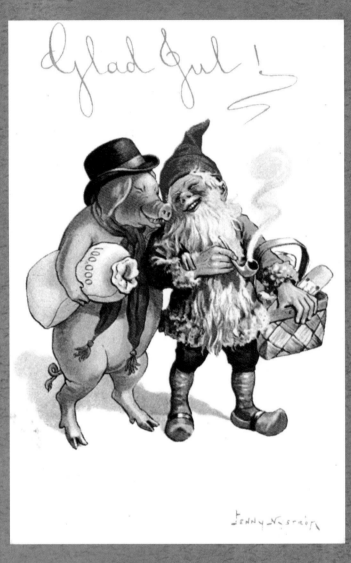

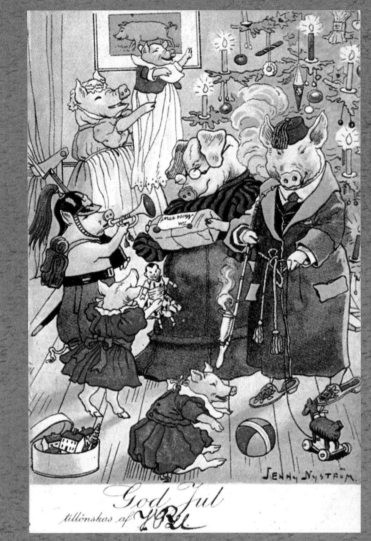

Jenny Nyström,
Axel Eliassons
Konstförlag,
Stockholm 1907.

Jenny Nyström,
Axel Eliassons
Konstförlag,
Stockholm 1904.

"Christmas cards on glossy stock indicate that the sender is a happy, pleasant, and very peaceful person who lacks the ability to concentrate." Hence, Christmas cards with velvet applications, to give special emphasis to the pattern, are selected by people who are particular about making an impression but could, according to experts, also be an indication of mistrust, jealousy, purposefulness, and obstinacy. Patterns where the color blue dominates are chosen for the most part by intellectuals with strong imagination. Darker colors are chosen by those with a sensitive nature. Red patterns are popular among women, the reason being that red is a strong force of attraction. Men who choose red Christmas cards are regarded as henpecked husbands or, at best, as dependent on others and longing for a motherly, dominant woman. Yellow Christmas cards indicate that the sender is an egotist or a recluse, with a longing for tenderness. Orange is selected by sociable individuals, and lilac by pompous people. "'Funny' Christmas cards are generally sent by people who are not very funny themselves." Now what does a card with a Christmas pig say about the sender?

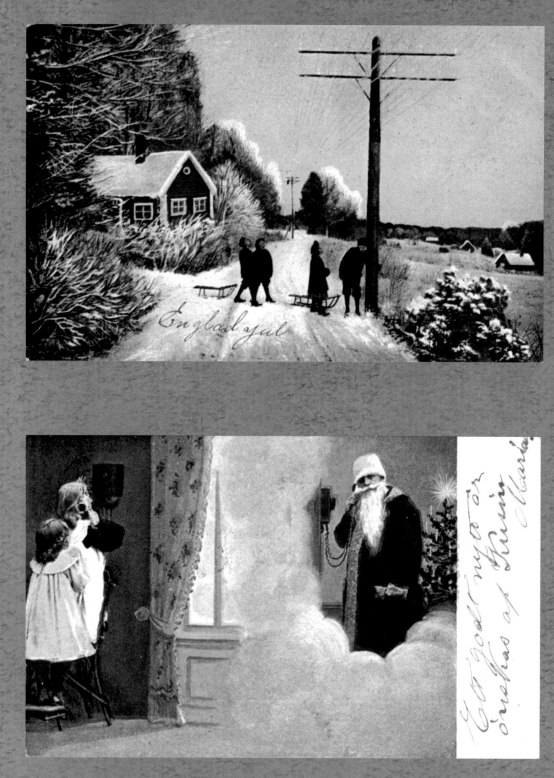

Axel Eliassons
Konstförlag,
Stockholm around
1906.

A card from a
series entitled "St.
Nicolaus,"
K.V.i.B. 1905–10.

Christmas Greetings When the first Christmas cards made an appearance, three quarters of the population lived in the countryside. The cards grew in popularity in step with a large-scale migration from the countryside to the cities. Or to America. However painful this process was, it was important to give it a positive spin, especially to those left behind, and the best way to do this was with a postcard. Cards were convenient because they only left room for a short message. It was cheap; the card cost five öre and the postage four öre. These factors together created a veritable postcard craze all year-round but especially at Christmas and New Year. Initially, Christmas and New Year's cards were delivered on the actual days. Cards that were mailed well in advance were sorted and kept in special boxes. There are many stories of invitation cards being mistakenly sorted as Christmas cards to the annoyance of hosts and hostesses.

Telegraphy and Telephony Eventually, the need for speed gave birth to telegraphy to be followed later by telephony. There were not many Christmas and New Year's greetings exchanged by telegram, but the Christmas card artists were quick to introduce these modernities in their motifs. Children listening to the faint sound of the telephone lines, illustrates a belief in the future that was universal at this time. There may not initially have been many telephone lines leading into the cottages, but you can be sure that the telephone had become a must-have for the next generation.

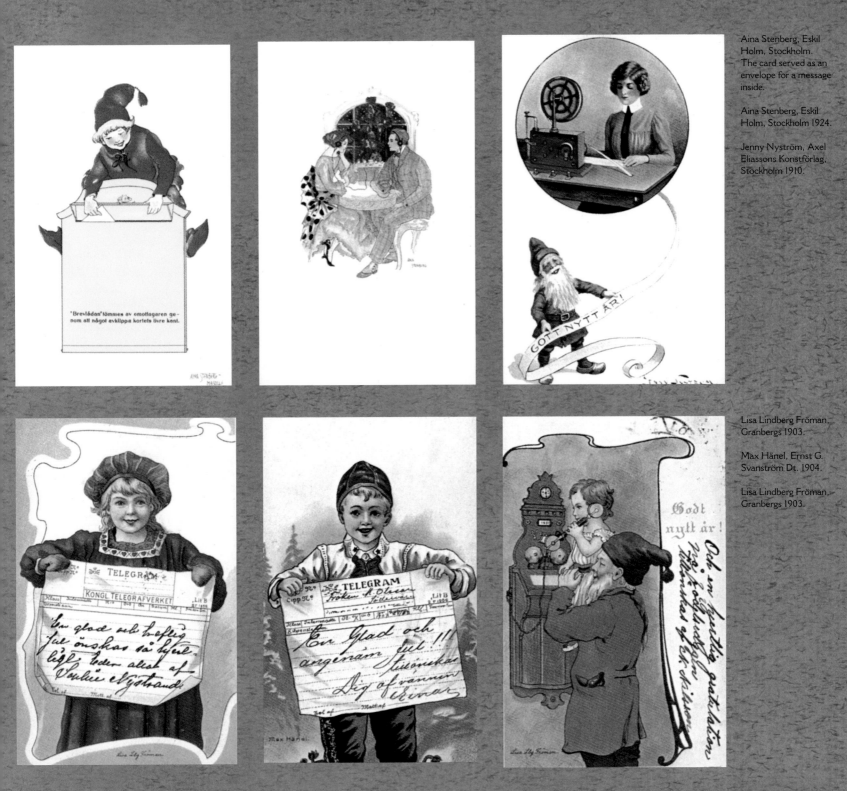

Aina Stenberg, Eskil Holm, Stockholm. The card served as an envelope for a message inside.

Aina Stenberg, Eskil Holm, Stockholm 1924.

Jenny Nyström, Axel Eliassons Konstförlag, Stockholm 1910.

Lisa Lindberg Fröman, Granbergs 1903.

Max Hänel, Ernst G. Svanström Dt. 1904.

Lisa Lindberg Fröman, Granbergs 1903.

Jenny Nyström,
Axel Eliassons
Konstförlag,
Stockholm 1908.

Jenny Nyström,
Axel Eliassons
Konstförlag,
Stockholm.

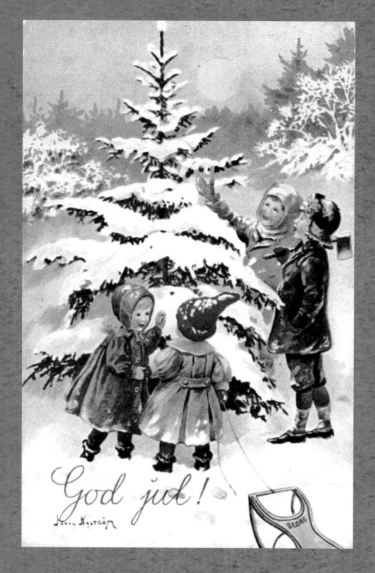

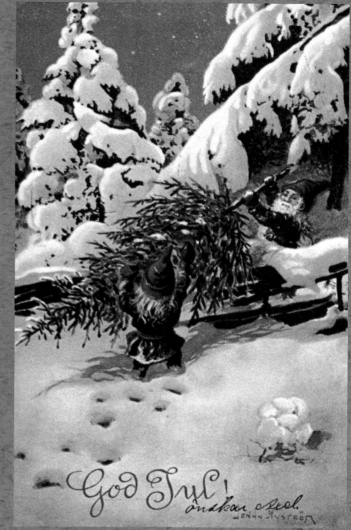

The Christmas Tree   The Christmas tree became commonplace in Sweden through its depiction on Christmas cards by Jenny Nyström and other artists. In really old Christmas cards the "continental" Santa, St. Nicholas, arrives with gifts for the nice children and twigs for the naughty. As a reminder of this, children were often given a twig in a jug of water that would blossom as Christmas neared. Later on, it became customary to decorate the twig with apples, gingerbread cookies, and candles. The step from twigs to Christmas trees was not a big one. The Christmas tree, like many other Christmas customs, was a German import.

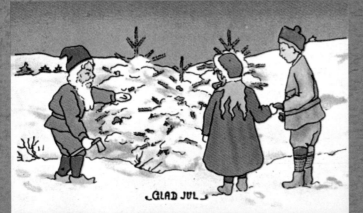

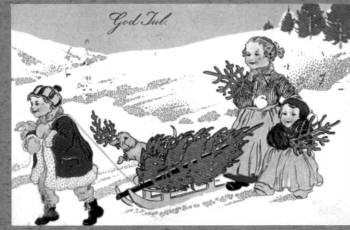

Anonymous.

Anonymous, P.F.B. 1906. The card was addressed to a passenger onboard the steamship Prins Gustaf.

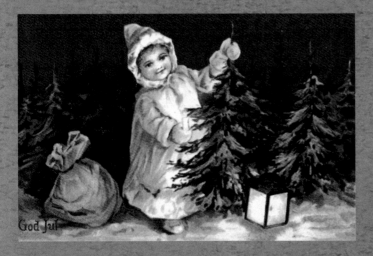

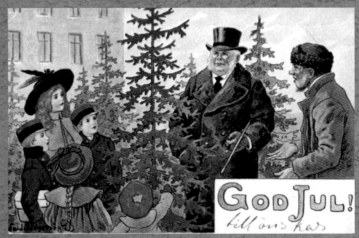

Anonymous German card from 1905–10.

Jenny Nyström, Axel Eliassons Konstförlag, Stockholm.

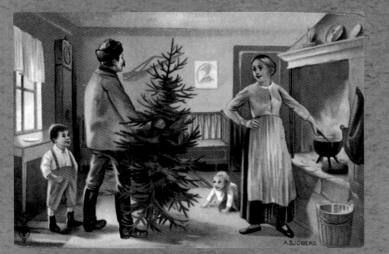

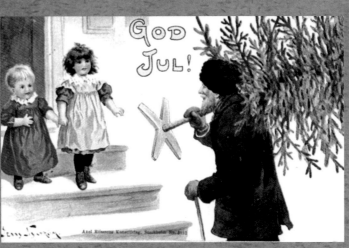

A. Sjöberg, Tullbergs Konstindustri AB 1896.

Jenny Nyström, Axel Eliassons Konstförlag, Stockholm 1909.

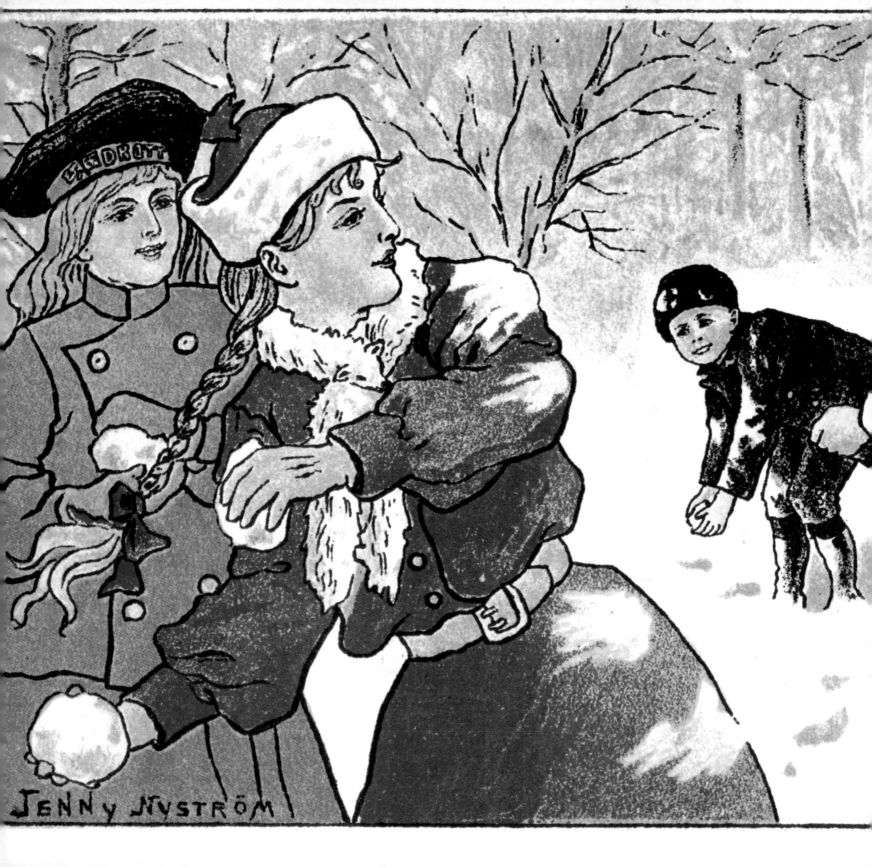

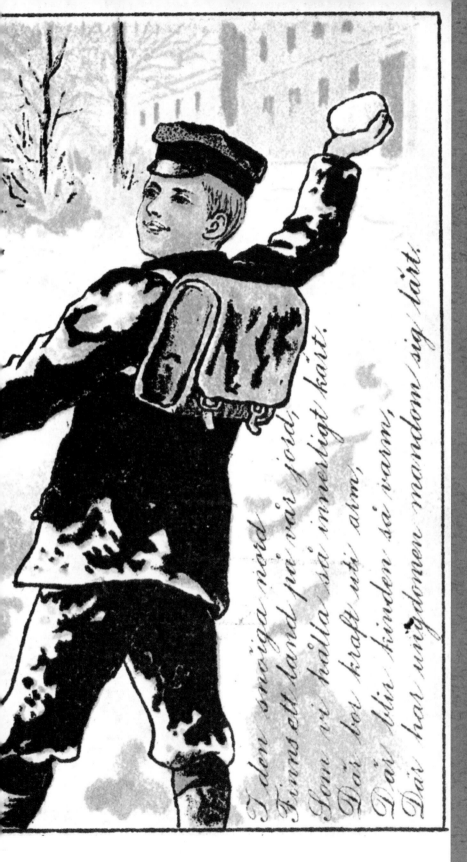

I den snöiga nord
Finns ett land på vår jord,
Som vi hålla så innerligt kärt.
Där får kraft uti arm,
Där blir kinden så varm,
Där har ungdomen mandom sig lärt.

God Jul!

Anonymous German card
printed in Saxony.

Outdoors   In the olden days, the snow always lay
invitingly white and unspoiled right up to the doorstep.
Christmas was a time for outdoor fun that included
tobogganing, skating, skiing, and sledding. Adults and
children alike made snowmen, snow lanterns, and
fortresses, and threw snowballs at each other. Santa was
not spared.

Jenny Nyström,
John Fröbergs
Förlag.

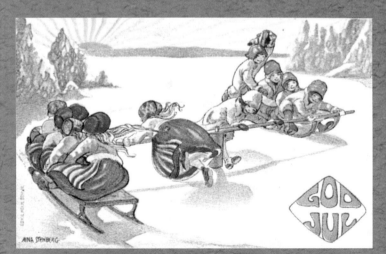

"Snowball card"
by Jenny Nyström,
Eskil Holm,
Stockholm.

"Miniature card" by
Aina Stenberg, Eskil
Holm, Stockholm.

"Tip-top-card" by
Aina Stenberg, Eskil
Holm, Stockholm.

Opposite page:

Jenny Berg 1916.

J.N.
(Jenny Nyström)
without the
publisher's name,
circa 1902.

28

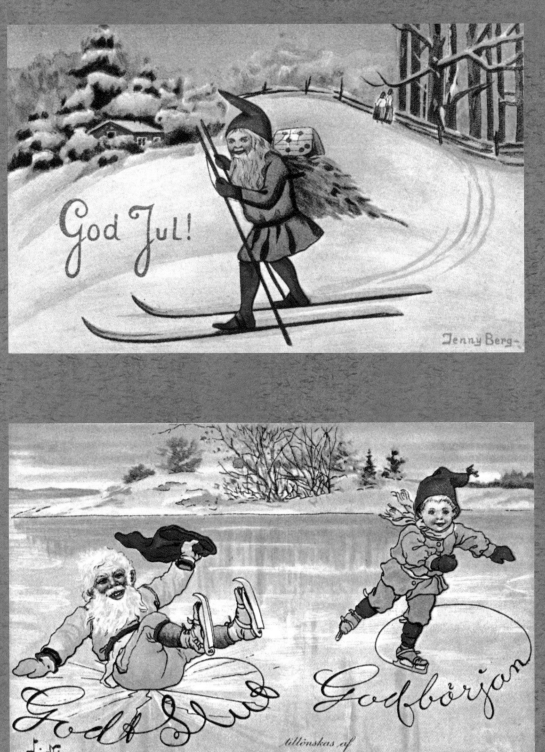

God Jul!

Jenny Berg

Godt Slut Godbörjan

tillönskas af

Winter Amusements

Snowball Cards   Irregularly shaped Christmas cards have always been popular. The snowball inspired Jenny Nyström to create a collection of "snowball cards" in the early 1900s. The inventive Aina Stenberg, who designed the depicted "tip-top-card" and "miniature card," also made a few cards with mechanisms. These were all echoes of the 19th-century penchant for imitations and fantastic materials and punched-out shapes. The motif was secondary and often more of an ornament added to accentuate the material. These cards were expensive to make and required an envelope, and they disappeared when the simple and standardized postcards became the norm. In later years, the expensive, dressed-up cards made a comeback as folded cards have overtaken postcards in popularity. The fold was originally introduced to make it easier to showcase Christmas cards on mantelpieces in British and American homes.

The World's Largest Christmas Card   Among the most unusual Christmas cards ever sent was the one received by the Prince of Wales in 1929. A small grain of rice contained not only the address but also a greeting and a picture of a car. The world's largest Christmas card was mailed in 1968. It was six miles long, weighed two tons, and was a greeting from soldiers who had returned from the Vietnam War to their comrades still serving in the war. It was delivered in the form of a paper roll by a specially chartered plane.

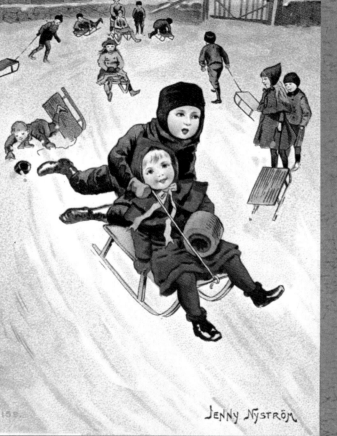

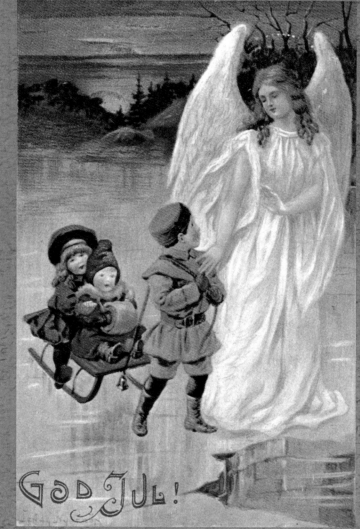

Jenny Nyström,
Axel Eliassons
Konstförlag,
Stockholm 1906.

Jenny Nyström,
Axel Eliassons
Konstförlag,
Stockholm 1906.

Card Series A Christmas card artist has to design four to ten different cards each spring for that year's production. The photographers that the card producers employed had to produce as many possible motifs in a single day. They really had to make full use of the scanty ideas, models, and settings they had at hand. It is therefore not unusual to see the same man drink to the New Year first with a blonde, then with a brunette, and so on. Series of two to ten cards with a short story were also produced. The "erotic cards" at the turn of the century were also sold as collectors' series. The cards with motifs of an advancing flirtation, exploited with a great deal of sensitivity the erotic charge in tobogganing, swinging, or other couple situations outside the bedroom.

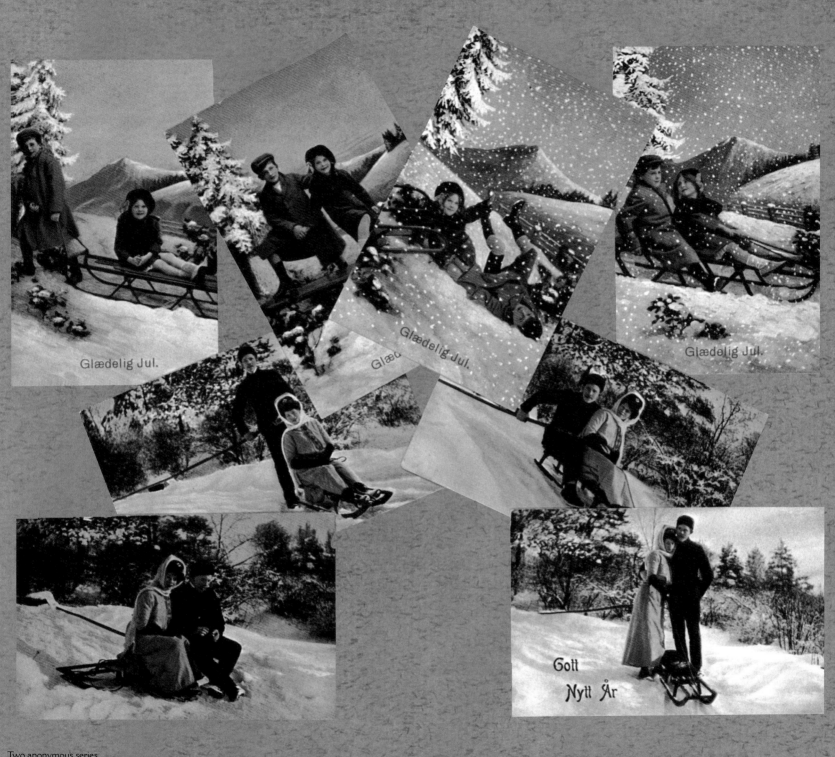

Glædelig Jul.

Glædelig Jul.

Glæd...

Glædelig Jul.

Gott Nytt År

Two anonymous series
of German cards.

Hildur Söderberg,
Granbergs.

Hildur Söderberg,
Granbergs.

Proessdorf,
accompanying
the *Julhälsning*
magazine from
Nordiska Förlaget
in Stockholm 1913.

Jenny Nyström,
Eskil Holm,
Stockholm 1905.

Anna Palm de Rosa,
Eskil Holm 1905.

A.H., Granbergs
1925.

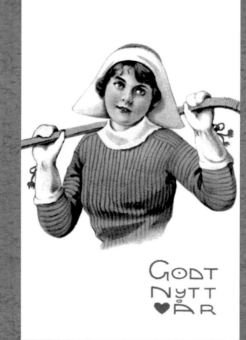

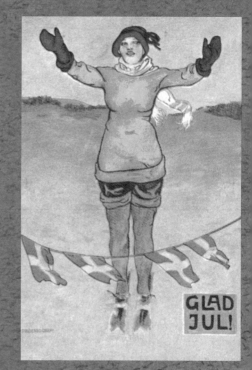

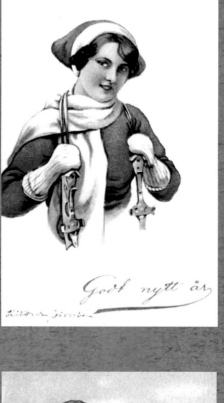

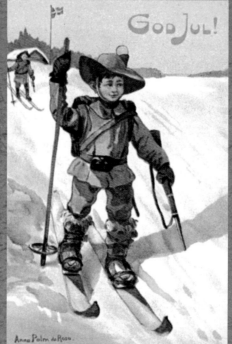

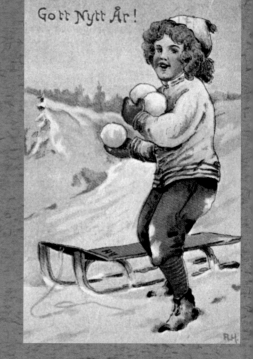

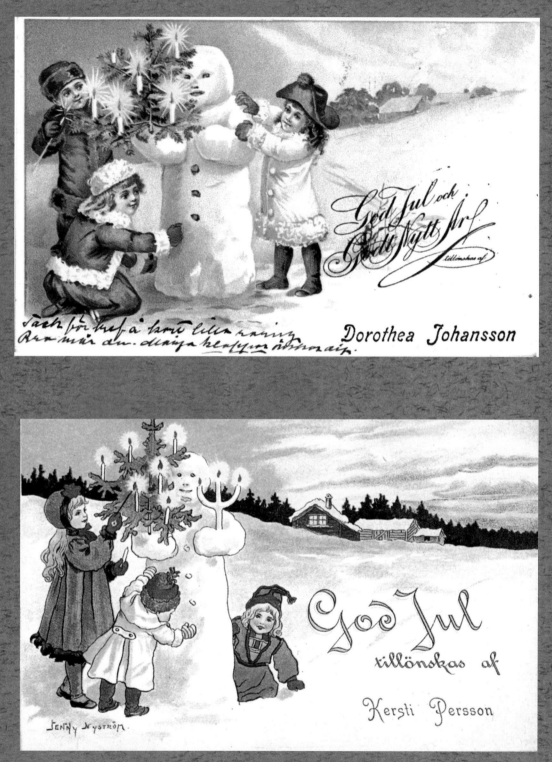

Anonymous 1903.

Jenny Nyström,
Fröbergs 1902–1904.

Dorothea Johansson

God Jul
tillönskas af

Kersti Persson

Child Motifs   Christmas is above all a holiday for children. It is also through children that Christmas becomes more meaningful for adults. Jenny Nyström loved to paint children. In her portrayal of her son Curt and his friends, there is an expression of innocence, goodness, and happiness. There are no naughty or troublesome children on Christmas cards. And that is why we can't help loving them. They live in the elucidated shimmer we want to remember Swedish own childhood in.

Mature Beauties   The children that are portrayed outdoors are more natural than those in the rather stuffy, interior scenes. It is also outdoors that we encounter young adults—who seem to be proscribed inside. The three young beauties are unique and could probably only have been depicted outdoors and in connection with a sport.

Anna Palm de Rosa   The young skier in the "landstorm" uniform, with the Swedish flag in the background, was popular in 1905. The card was painted by Anna Palm, the artist most closely connected with the early Swedish postcards. Her watercolors, with different city motifs, are among the most sought-after by Swedish and foreign postcard collectors. Anna Palm, born in 1859, was the daughter of a landscape painter. She added "de Rosa" to her name after her marriage to an Italian officer.

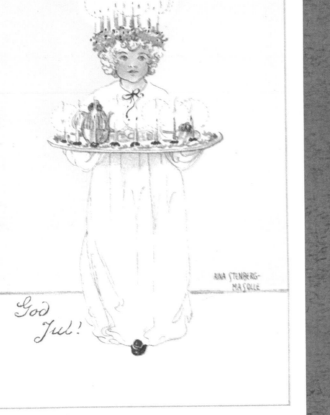

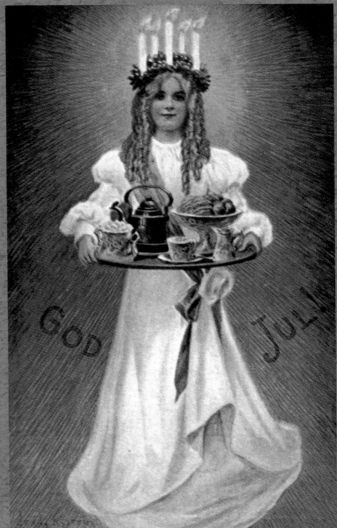

Aina Stenberg-MasOlle, Eskil Holm, Stockholm.

Jenny Nyström, Axel Eliassons Konstförlag, Stockholm 1910.

Leading up to Christmas

Lucia   Several Nobel laureates have been frightened when they have been woken by the beautiful song of the candle-bearing Lucia in their room at Stockholm's Grand Hotel on the morning of December 13. The coffee and the saffron bun have been good compensations for the rude awakening. Lucia is the only uniquely Swedish Christmas tradition. The first Lucia was likely an angel with wings and a crown with lighted candles as a halo in an end-of-term Christmas play. In earlier figures of Lucia, the wings are still on but the candles are on a tray. Adopted as a tradition by the upper class, Lucia spread to universities and schools before it evolved into a public Christmas celebration that is a must at every place of work and school all over Sweden on December 13. The tradition became official when *Stockholms-Tidningen* in 1927 turned it into more of a pageant. The export of Lucia has also been very successful.

Lucifer   Lucia has been adorned by the legend of Santa Lucia as well as the Lucia song which, in the original Italian version, is all about the port of Naples. In medieval times, the night of Lucia was the longest of the year and therefore favored by the devil and his followers. Lucia, and its much older predecessor, Lusse, have, in all likelihood, as strong a connection with Lucifer—the devil, as with Lux—light, in Latin. The shape of the saffron Lucia bun (*lussekatt*) probably stems from a cat being one of the many shapes that the devil could take on when he visited mortals.

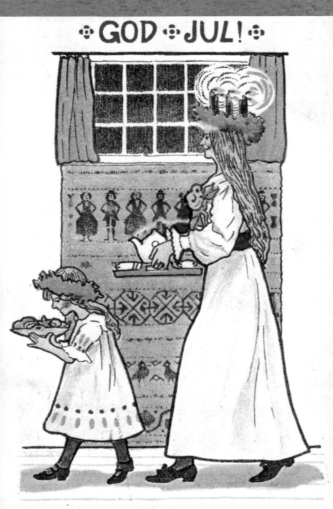

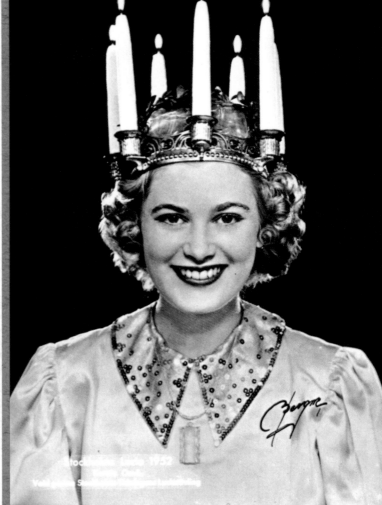

Anonymous 1912.

Kerstin Ornö, the Stockholm Lucia in 1952. She was chosen in a competition in *StockholmsTidningen* and photographed by Bergne.

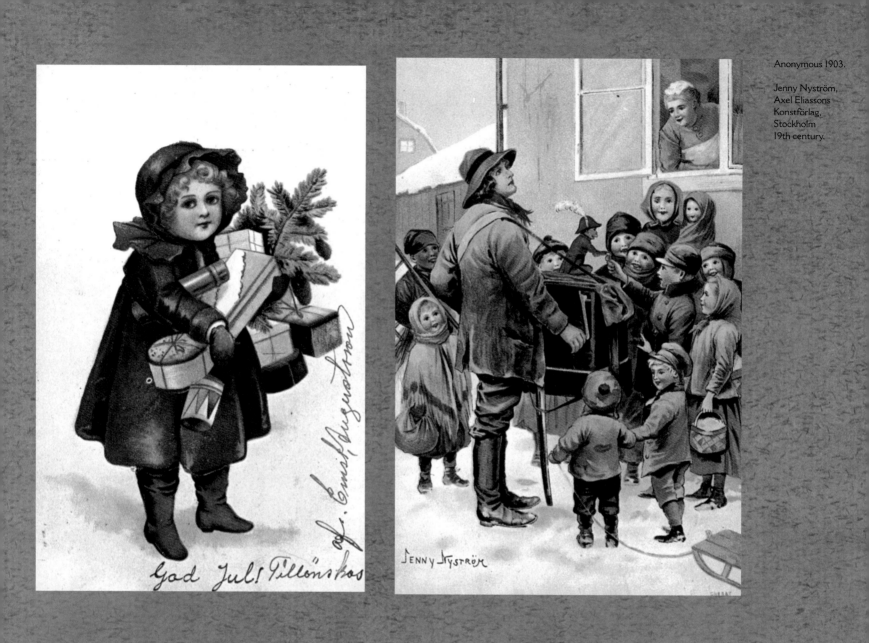

Anonymous 1903.

Jenny Nyström,
Axel Eliassons
Konstförlag,
Stockholm
19th century.

God Jul! Tillönskos

JENNY NYSTRÖM

Tomas Day   December 21, Tomas Day, was a traditional market day. In the past it was a day the "Christmas peace" set in. Anybody who continued to work after this day could be befallen by the most terrible mishaps. The only ones who were allowed to work were the pastor and all supernatural beings. On Tomas Day, everybody dressed up in their Sunday best for a visit to the closest market. But before leaving the house, there had to be a traditional sip of the Christmas beer which by now had fermented to perfection. One of the items that was to be purchased at the market was aquavit, that is if it had not already been brewed at home. The market visit was by tradition a "wet" affair and the day was popularly called "Tomas Drunkard" (Tomas Fylletunna).

Christmas Market   At the Stortorget market in Stockholm, there were 95 vendors in 1838. Apart from the trinkets and fancy goods booths, there were bakers, sheet metal workers, bookbinders, brush-makers, jewelers, hatters, toy sellers and soap makers,

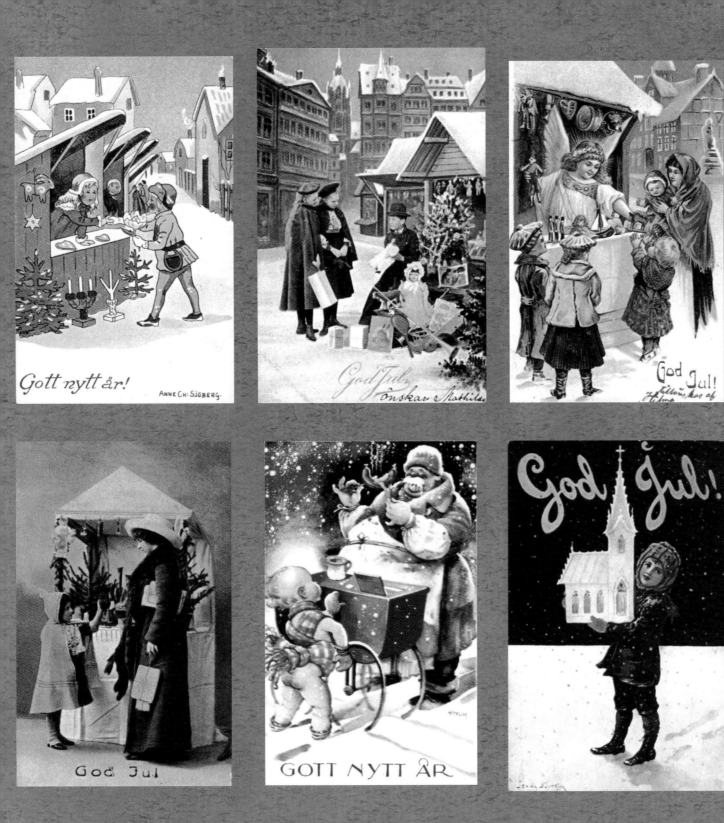

Jenny Nyström,
Axel Eliassons
Konstförlag,
Stockholm 1908.
The card has a
greeting in Finnish.

Anonymous,
Ferdinand Hey'l,
Stockholm 1900s.

Jenny Nyström
1906 (no publisher's
name).

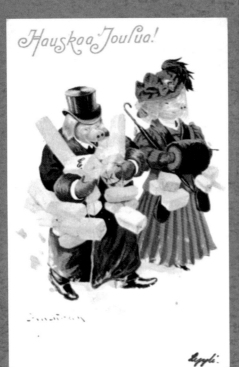

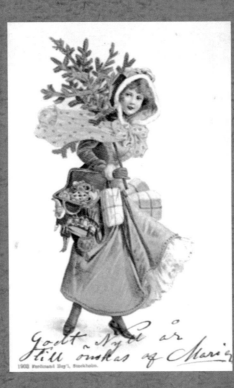

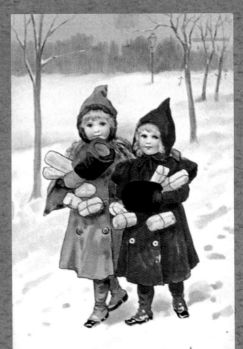

Jenny Nyström,
Axel Eliassons
Konstförlag,
Stockholm 1905.

V. Schonberg,
Svenska Litografiska
Anstalten.

Jenny Nyström,
Axel Eliassons
Konstförlag,
Stockholm.

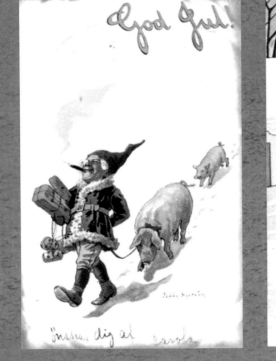

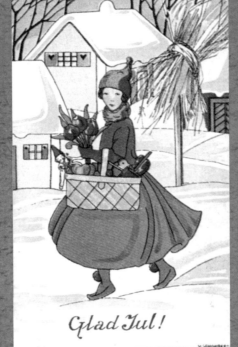

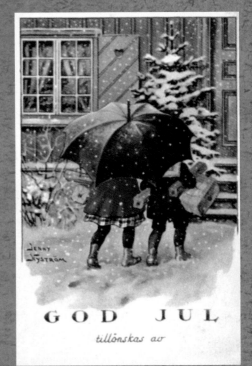

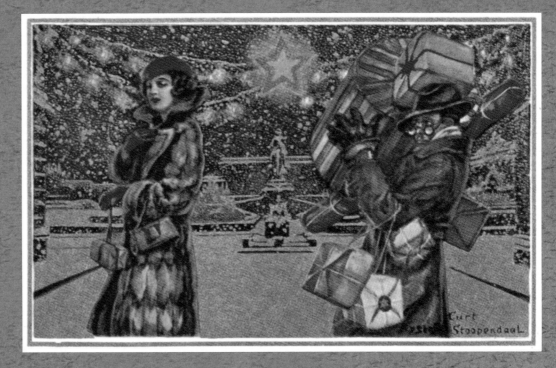

Curt Nyström
Stoopendaal,
Axel Eliassons
Konstförlag,
Stockholm 1907.

Jenny Nyström,
Axel Eliassons
Konstförlag,
Stockholm 1925.

instrument makers, basket weavers, and many more. The market gave the farmer an opportunity to make some money from the products of the farm and spend it on all kinds of Christmas specialties. The grocer had fruits and other delicacies that were impossible to get during the rest of the year. There was a great choice of Christmas tree ornaments and decorations for the home. There were Christmas stars made of paper or straw to hang at windows, and textile hangings to decorate walls and ceilings. Many Christmas card artists also produced an annual paper version of the hanging. Plaster of Paris churches that could be illuminated were highly treasured. There was, of course, no lack of all kinds of carnies, carousing and general merrymaking at the markets. Children were treated to cotton candy or hot dogs from Helge Artelius' impressive booth.

The Commercial Christmas   These cards are a reflection of the modest beginnings of the commercial Christmas. The Christmas markets really only sold such goods that could not be made at home. The upper middle class attire of those carrying the parcels tells us that the purchase of such goods was the reserved privilege of but a few. The purchases were normally carried home by porters, so the parcels on the cards are more a symbol of the merry abundance of Christmas than a real life situation.

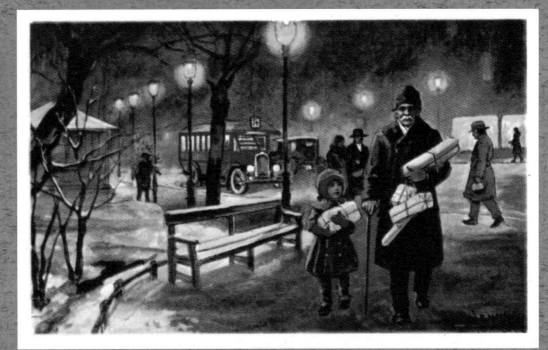

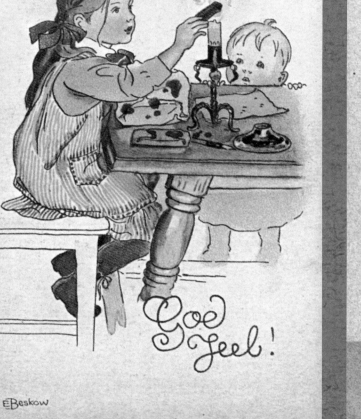

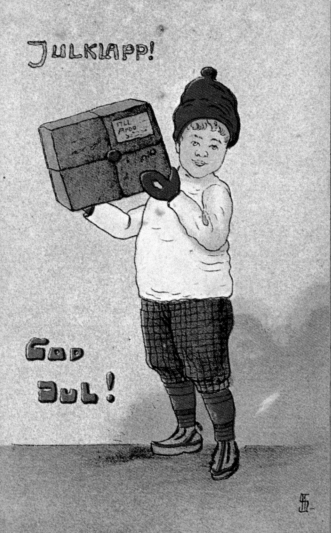

Elsa Beskow,
Axel Eliassons
Konstförlag,
Stockholm 1913.

The signature THS,
Åhlén & Holm.

Elsa Beskow   In the book *Petter och Lottas Jul* by Elsa Beskow, we read about how Lotta crocheted and sewed all her Christmas gifts while Petter made his from wood. Afterward, they packaged their gifts in lots of paper and sealed them, so that there would be lots of suspense when the parcels were opened. Lotta looks a lot like the little girl with the stick of sealing wax on the Christmas card above.

Elsa Beskow was an artist, painter, and author who created the classic Swedish illustrated children's book. When she, around the turn of the century, became the art teacher at the Whitlock School in Stockholm, she started illustrating Christmas magazines. Later, between 1912 and 1914, she also created lots of beautiful Christmas cards.

Aina Stenberg,
Eskil Holm,
Stockholm 1939.

H Söderberg,
Svenska
Litografiska AB,
Stockholm.

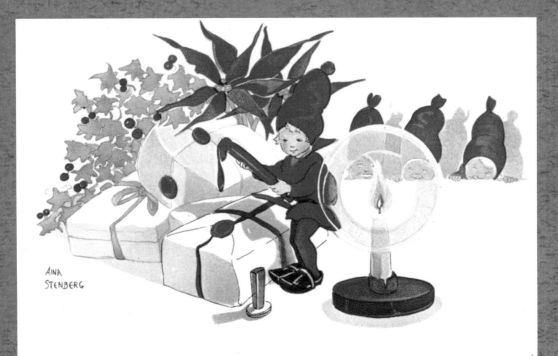

Sealing Christmas Gifts The smell of the bright red sealing wax is, for many Swedes, the ultimate smell of Christmas. But these days, most Christmas gifts are packed by store assistants when they are bought, and the intricate packing, the wax sparkling in the candle, the spitting on the seal and the satisfaction of achieving a perfect seal are becoming a thing of the past. And not many Christmas rhymes are written any longer either.

An Evening of Preparations In the past a family, sometimes joined by farm employees and their families, would gather together for a "stay-up-evening." This was on a normal work night and did not really have anything special to do with Christmas. The radio program "Only Mother is Awake," hosted by Maud Reuterswärd, popularized the idea of a "stay-up-evening" before Christmas when the family gathered around the kitchen table to pack Christmas gifts, make ornaments, and prepare toffee and other goodies.

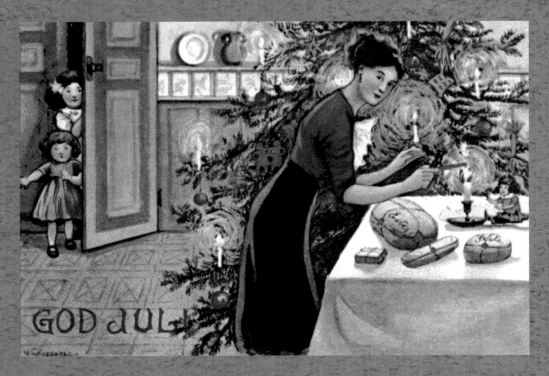

G. Stoopendaal,
Calegi Sto.

Isaac Grünewald,
Axel Eliassons
Konstförlag,
Stockholm.

Jenny Nyström,
Axel Eliassons
Konstförlag,
Stockholm.

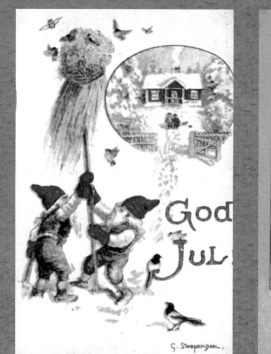

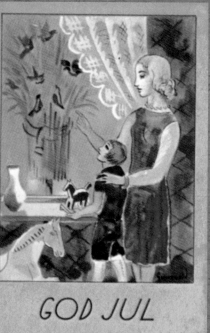

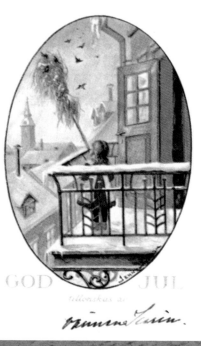

M. Hänel 1901.

Jenny Nyström,
Axel Eliassons
Konstförlag,
Stockholm 1925.

Anders Olsson,
AB Ingvar Larsson.

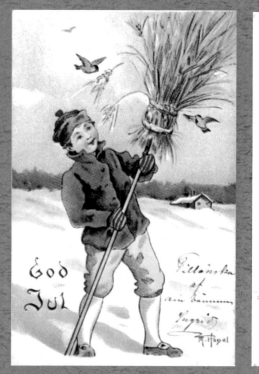

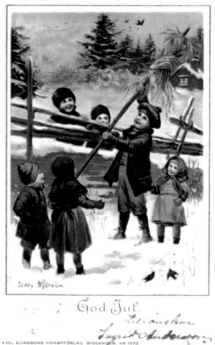

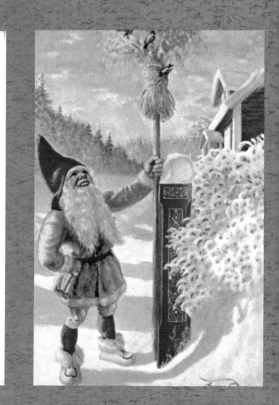

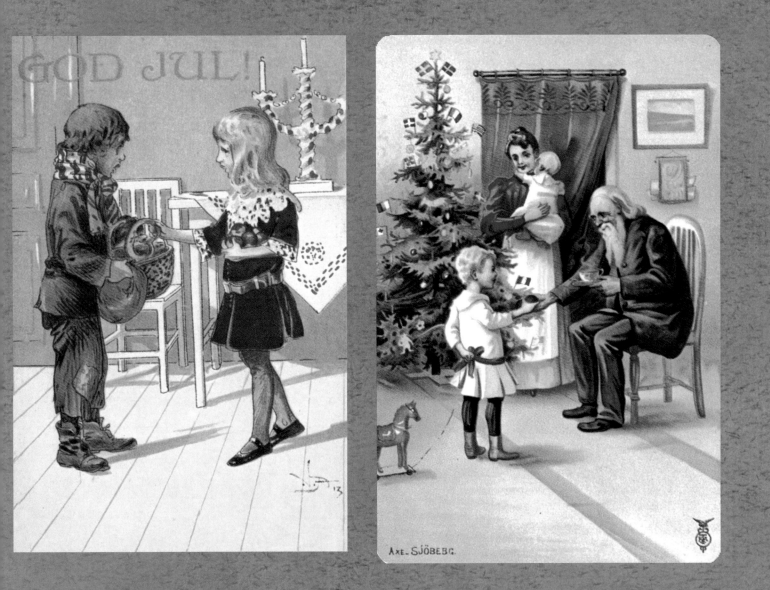

GOD JUL!

AXE. SJÖBEBG.

The Christmas Sheaf Christmas is a time when generosity toward both people and animals abounds. In the old days, every visitor was to be treated to food and drink, otherwise they would rob the home of Christmas. The sheaf, put out for the birds as another symbol of this benevolence, is a motif on numerous Christmas cards including one by the famous painter Isaac Grünewald. The sheaf is a remnant from heathen times when the spirit of the harvest was believed to remain in the last sheaf harvested. This sheaf was raised on a high stake in the yard to bless the family, the animals, the earth, and all worldly possessions.

Opposite page:

ID 1907.

Colored
photograph,
K.V.i.B.,
Köpenhamn 1903.

Anonymous 1902.

Anonymous,
Axel Eliassons
Konstförlag,
Stockholm 1909.

Anonymous photo,
RP.

G. Stoopendaal,
Nilssons
Ljustrycksanstalt,
Stockholm 1915.

G. Stoopendaal,
Nilssons
Ljustrycksanstalt,
Stockholm 1910.

Colored photograph
from Axel Eliassons
Konstförlag,
Stockholm.

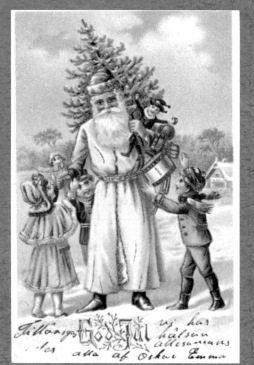

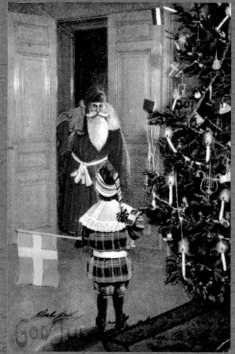

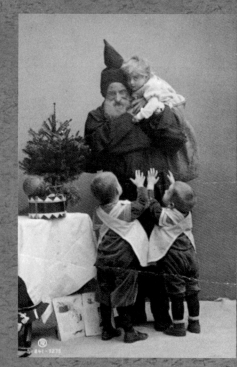

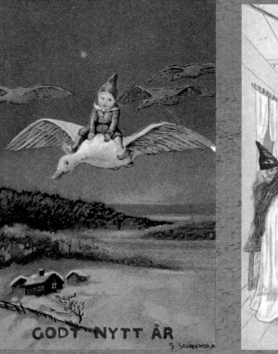

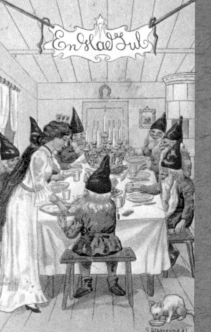

Come All Ye Santas

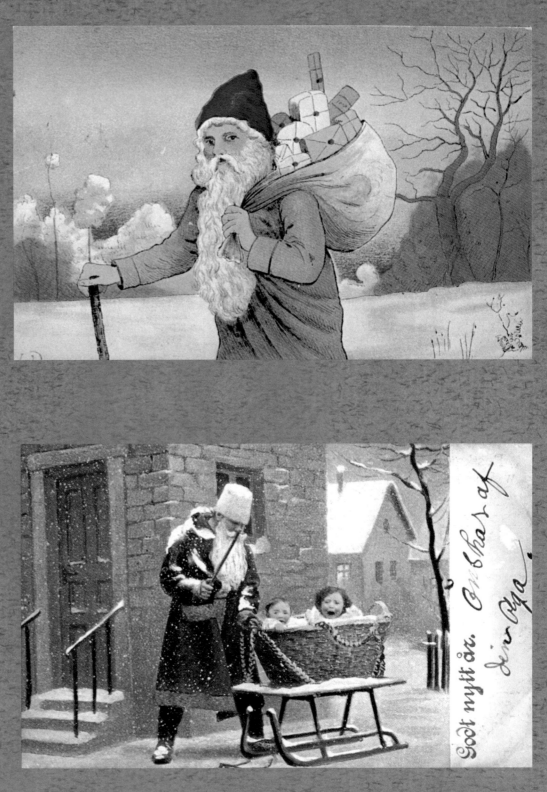

St. Nicholas   Older Santas look a lot like Greek priests. They are tall and grand with imposing beards. St. Nicholas was a bishop in Asia Minor in the year 300, who, after his death, became one of the most popular saints, especially with schools, children, and travelers. When his day was celebrated in Catholic schools on December 6, the good students got praise and presents from St. Nicholas while the bad students got a symbolic taste of the rod by the little devil figure that accompanied him. Eventually the two figures merged, but the question "Are there any good children here?" that all Swedish kids are asked by Santa, still serves as a reminder. Nicholas was so popular that he survived the reformation to become Sinterklaas in Holland and Santa Claus in the English-speaking world.

The Swedish Santa   The *jultomte* in Sweden is a mixture of St. Nicholas, other foreign Santa figures, and the *tomte* of Swedish folklore. He was a house spirit of Germanic origin, who brought the farm and its inhabitants luck, even if he had to steal it from the neighbors. Viktor Rydberg defined the tomte's character in the story *Little Vigg's Adventure on Christmas Eve*, in 1871, and ten years later in the poem *Tomten*. Jenny Nyström, who illustrated both the story and the poem, started combining Nicholas, the German Christmas man, Snow White's seven dwarfs, Kilian Zoll's first Swedish Santa in 1851, and all the other little gnomes to create the Swedish Santa.

Jenny Nyström,
Axel Eliassons
Konstförlag,
Stockholm 1912.

Jenny Nyström,
(no publisher's
name).

Jenny Nyström,
Axel Eliassons
Konstförlag,
Stockholm.

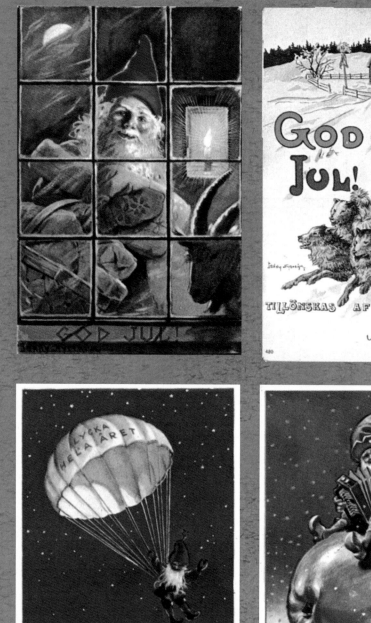

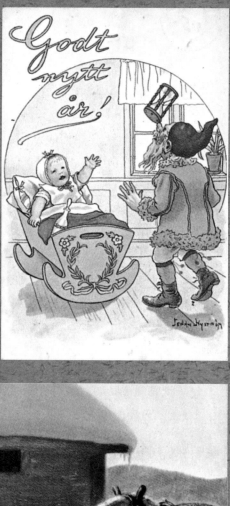

Jenny Nyström,
Axel Eliassons
Konstförlag,
Stockholm.

Curt Nyström
Stoopendaal,
Axel Eliassons
Konstförlag,
Stockholm.

Anders Olsson,
AB Ingvar Larson
Konstförlag.

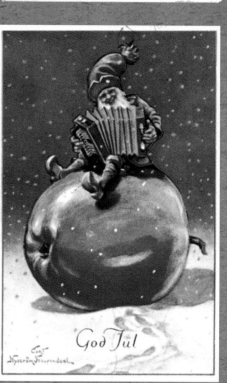

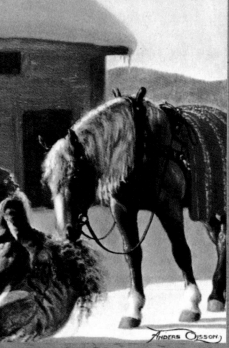

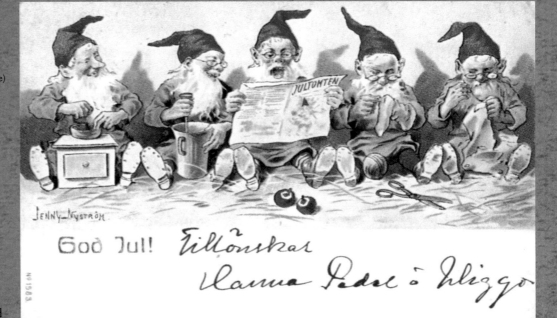

Jenny Nyström When the 17-year-old Jenny Nyström read *Little Vigg's Adventure on Christmas Eve* in *Handelstidningen* in 1871, she got so inspired that she proceeded to illustrate it. When the story was published as a book, it was Nyström's Santa drawings that were used even though the author Viktor Rydberg did not think that they matched his picture of Santa. When Jenny Nyström later illustrated the poem *Tomten*, she used her father as a model and a different type of Santa emerged. It was quite similar to Nyström's teacher Fredrik Wohlfart's Santas, but eventually got a profile of its own. All kinds of Santas of all ages emerged that were up to all kinds of things like cycling, driving cars. jumping with parachutes, or listening to the radio.

Jenny Nyström (1854–1946) had started a promising traditional artistic career as a portraitist and landscape painter. She studied at Konstakademien in Stockholm, in Munich and in Paris and, already in her youth, received the much-coveted Royal medal. But her serious painting at the easel has been completely overshadowed by her enormous production of illustrations and cards. For these, she has done literally thousands of clever variations of a limited number of Christmas motifs and motifs with children, a true testimony of her creativity. Many artists, including her son Curt Nyström Stoopendaal, followed her lead. The cards and small posters of the mother and son are sometimes hard to tell apart.

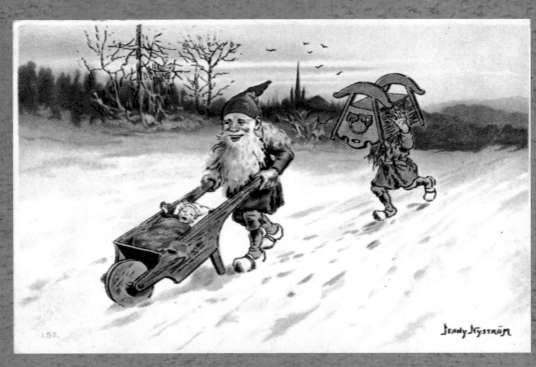

Aina Stenberg,
Eskil Holm,
Stockholm 1939
(72, 74, 76).

Aina Stenberg,
Eskil Holm,
Stockholm 1939
(64, 72, 73, 74, 76).

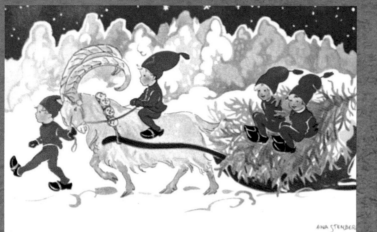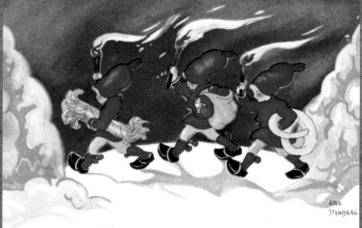

Aina Stenberg,
Eskil Holm,
Stockholm 1939
(64, 72, 73, 74, 76).

Aina Stenberg,
Eskil Holm,
Stockholm 1948.

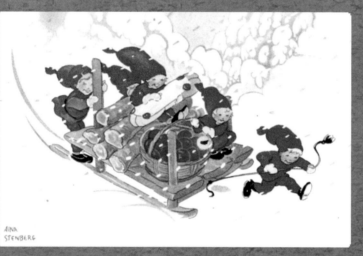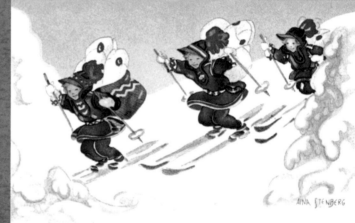

Aina Stenberg,
Eskil Holm,
Stockholm 1951
(78).

Aina Stenberg,
Eskil Holm,
Stockholm 1947
(75, 78).

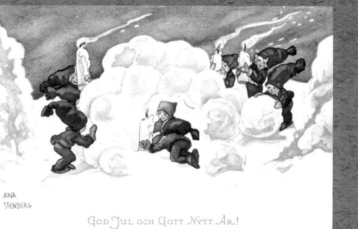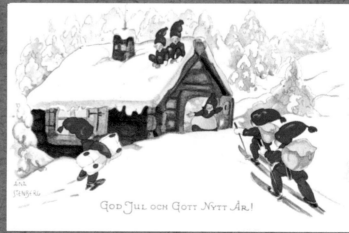

Aina Stenberg MasOlle   Jenny Nyström was undoubtedly the leading Christmas card artist with a naturalistic style, but when it comes to the decorative school, the foremost representative was unarguably Aina Stenberg. She varied two motifs to perfection on cards, runners, napkins, placement cards, posters, and advent calendars. Her signature small Santas and the beautiful "national cards," with colorful provincial costumes, were inspired by the summers and Christmases spent in the folkloristic province of Dalarna where Aina Stenberg's husband, painter Helmer MasOlle, grew up. Aina Stenberg painted a couple of thousand motifs, selling her first Christmas motif for one krona at the age of 18 and ending her painting career in her 90s when she was beginning to lose her eyesight. While Aina Stenberg's lead pencils were sharpened until they were like needles, her watercolors were soft and fresh. The effect of this was further enhanced as her cards were hand-lithographed in eight colors. Her motifs got simpler and cleaner as she aged.

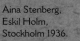

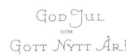

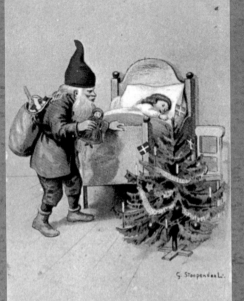

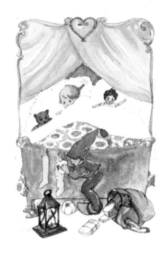

God Jul och Gott Nytt År

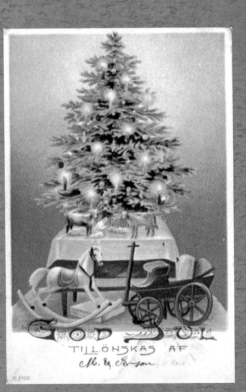

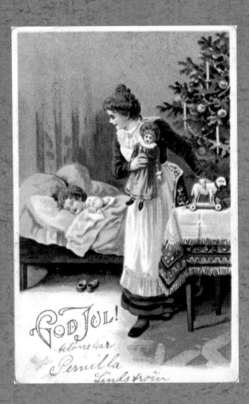

G. Stoopendaahl,
Carl Nilssons
Ljustrycksanstalt,
Stockholm.

Aina Stenberg,
Eskil Holm,
Stockholm 1957
(1978).

Anonymous 1905.

Anonymous 1906.

Haddon Sundblom   Curiously, the artist who gave the world its picture of Santa Claus, was not represented on a single Christmas card in Sweden. Haddon Sundblom, with Swedish-Finnish roots from the island of Åland, became a very successful commercial artist in Chicago. His first Santa Claus appeared in an advertisement in the *Saturday Evening Post* in 1931, and for the next 35 years he created new Santa ads each year for the Coca-Cola Company. Just as Jenny Nyström used her father as a model, Sundblom, who painted in the same classical style as Anders Zorn, based his Santa on a retired salesman who had the right build and "the wrinkles in his face all seemed to be happy wrinkles." When the salesman passed away, Haddon Sundblom used himself as a model because by then his broad, Nordic face also had the same kind of happy wrinkles. A Swedish kid's image of a Santa today may very well resemble the one Haddon Sundblom created for Coca-Cola, rather than a traditional tomte. But then there is a true Nordic connection hidden away in those wrinkles.

Little Santa   In North America and Great Britain, children get their gifts on the morning of Christmas Day. In Germany, children wake to find all their unwrapped gifts under the Christmas tree. In Sweden, many children get a few small gifts, from Little Santa, in their stockings on the morning of Christmas Eve. This keeps them busy until the real Santa arrives after dinner. Yes, to this day, almost all Swedish children get a visit from a flesh-and-blood Santa on Christmas Eve—a uniquely Swedish tradition. In days of old, many children also got a gift in advance on Tomas Day, which was celebrated as "Little Christmas" with a pre-taste of all the food and drink that was waiting to be consumed on Christmas Eve.

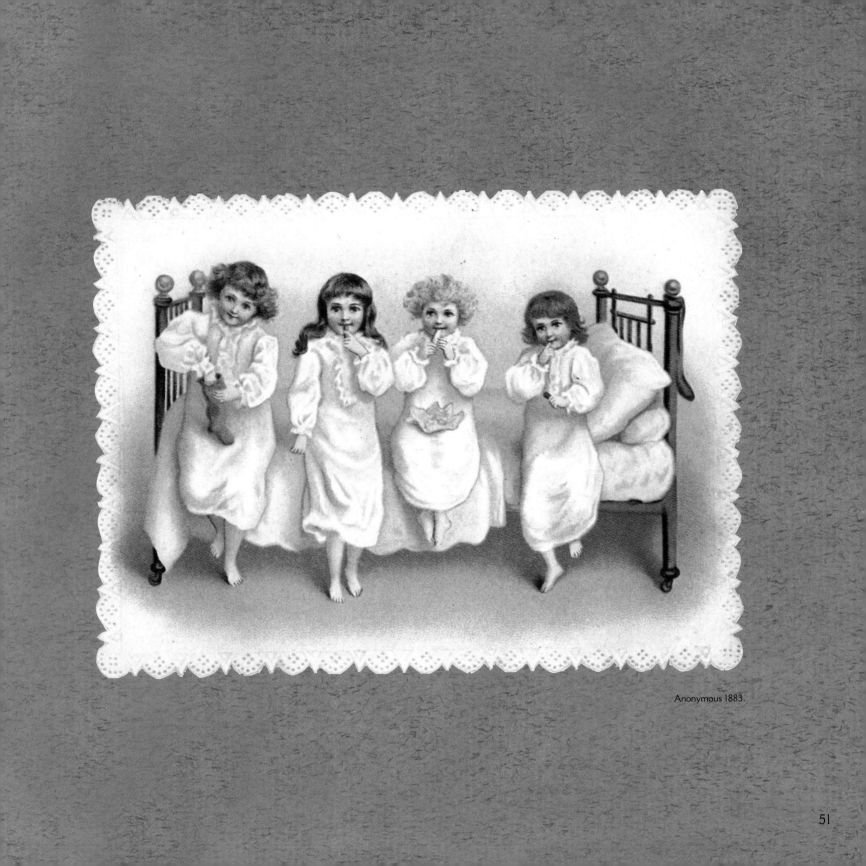

Anonymous 1883.

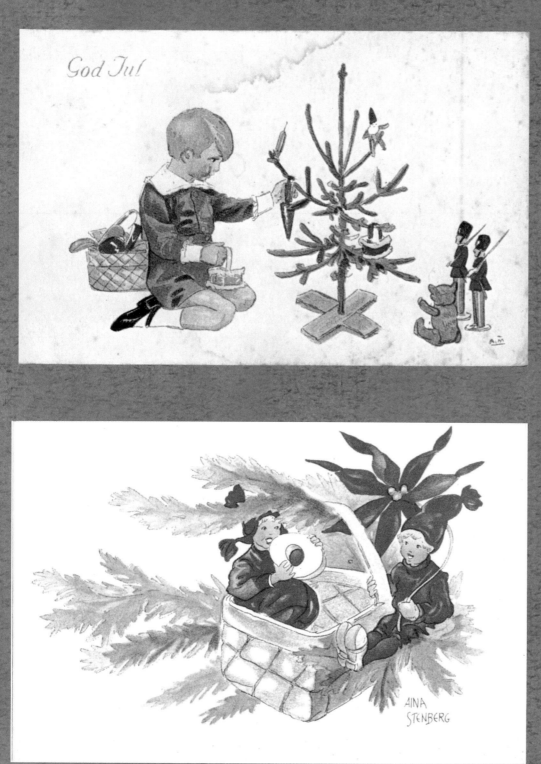

God Jul

AINA STENBERG

Christmas At Last

Decorating the Christmas Tree Before the Christmas tree became common in Sweden, around the turn of the last century, it was customary, in the countryside, to decorate a tall candle holder. Made out of wood, it was covered in red and green paper before apples and candles were added. When the spruces took over, they were decorated quite differently by the various social stratifications. A farm laborer's Christmas tree could, as its only decoration, have cotton wool meant to look like snow on the branches. A tree in a wealthy home in the city, meanwhile, would be covered with paper-wrapped candies, marzipan figurines, cookies, apples, birds of glass, flags, candles and hearts of plaited paper holding nuts, or other goodies. Figurines in the form of dogs, cats, bells, children, and flower baskets were often hung from a loop of thread. Made out of sugar and chalk by the local baker, the figurines were hard as stone and hardly edible, to the disappointment of all children. The confectioner's marzipan figurines, on the other hand, often made their way straight to the candy buffet. The tree had to be topped with a flag or a star. The popularity of the flags posed a real problem for Christmas card producers. It was, for instance, impossible to sell pictures of trees decorated with Swedish flags to the Danes. The artists solved this dilemma by either drawing all the Nordic flags on the tree or, at times, by changing the flags for each individual country. The spirit of internationalism on Christmas cards today is quite obviously a surrender to commercial considerations, with a single motif serving as many markets as possible.

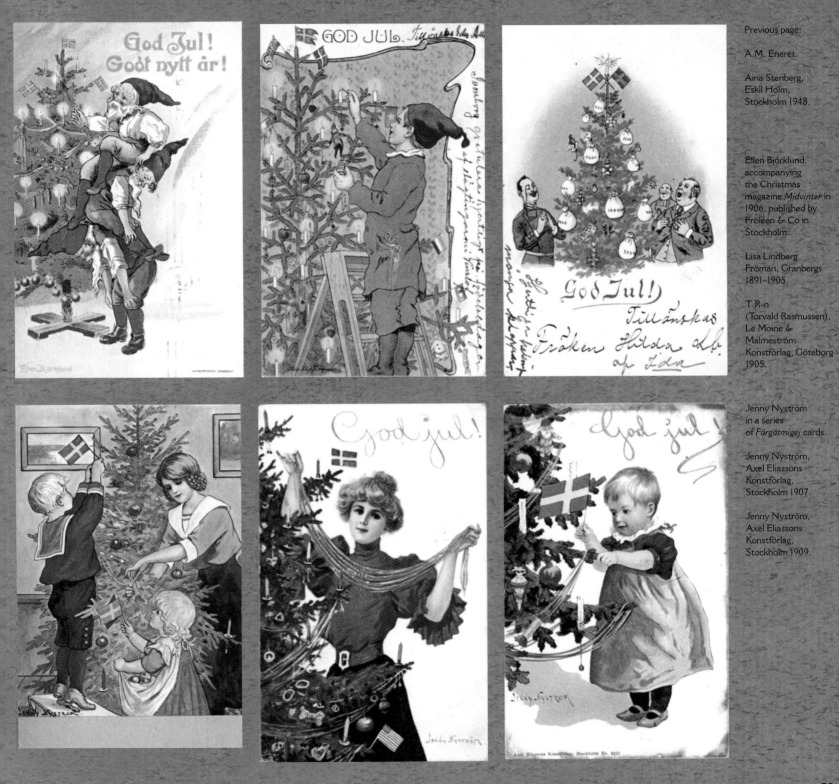

Previous page:

A.M. Eneret.

Aina Stenberg, Eskil Holm, Stockholm 1948.

Ellen Björklund, accompanying the Christmas magazine *Midvinter* in 1906, published by Fröléen & Co in Stockholm.

Lisa Lindberg Fröman, Granbergs 1891–1905.

T R-n (Torvald Rasmussen), Le Moine & Malmeström Konstförlag, Göteborg 1905.

Jenny Nyström in a series of *Förgätmigej* cards.

Jenny Nyström, Axel Eliassons Konstförlag, Stockholm 1907.

Jenny Nyström, Axel Eliassons Konstförlag, Stockholm 1909.

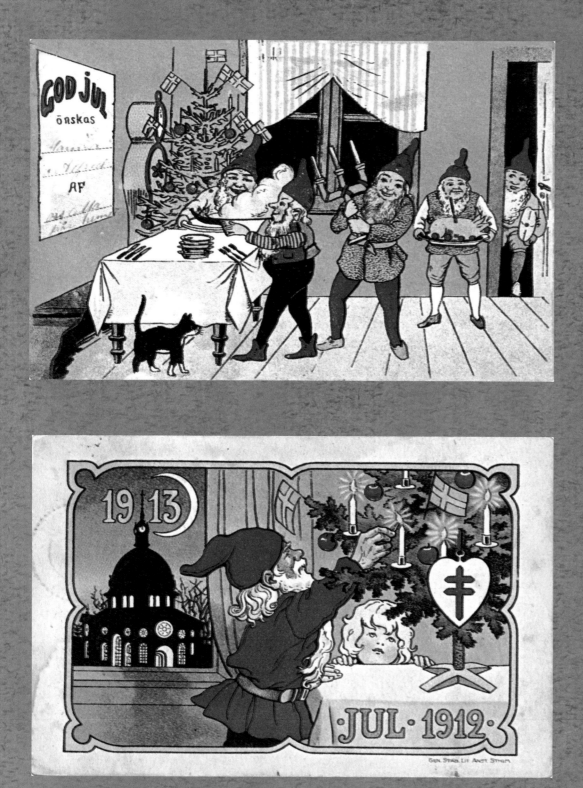

Anonymous 1905–10.

Jenny Nyström.
A card showing
the Svenska
Nationalförsamlingen
mot Tuberkolos
campaign sticker
of 1912.

The Final Preparations When the Christmas tree was decorated and little Christmas posters covered as many of the walls and ceilings as possible, the floors were covered with straw. In urban areas, the preferred covering was spruce branches, but eventually the insurance companies pulled the brakes on this custom. Not only did the house have to be spic and span, people also had to be squeaky clean for Christmas. For many, this involved the first and last full bath of the year. On farms, everybody took a bath in order according to their family ranking, in the same water. After the bath, new clothes, or clothes that had been part of the big Christmas wash, were put on. When this monumental task was completed, it had to be topped off with several shots of aquavit. Bring on Christmas!

All Decorated and Ready Christmas cards never depict all the nitty-gritty work involved in the Christmas preparations. Everything is always magically decorated and perfect. We see the master of the house light the last candle on the perfectly dressed tree while children and adults look on starry-eyed. If it ever looks like a lot of work, there is always a little Santa ready to step in and help. And if the Santas are otherwise occupied, there are helpful angels, on older cards, ready to lend a hand. The guardian angels were let loose by a papal decree in 1883 so that they could fly and help out in all kinds of situations.

54

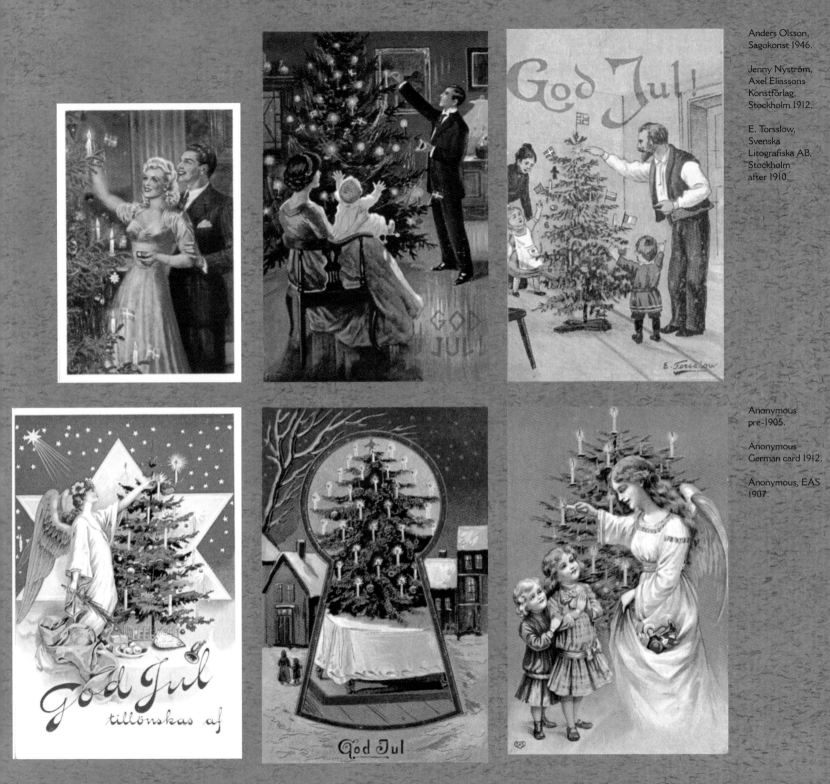

Jenny Nyström,
Axel Eliassons
Konstförlag,
Stockholm 1905.

Jenny Nyström,
Axel Eliassons
Konstförlag,
Stockholm 1906.

Jenny Nyström,
without any name
of publisher.

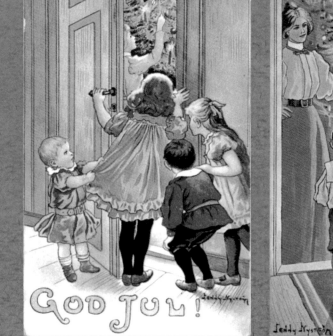

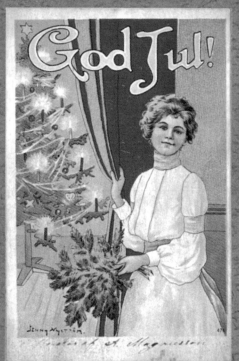

Anders Olsson,
Ingvar Larsson
Konst AB.

Jenny Nyström,
Axel Eliassons
Konstförlag,
Stockholm 1913.

Anonymous,
Axel Eliassons
Konstförlag,
Stockholm.

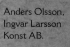

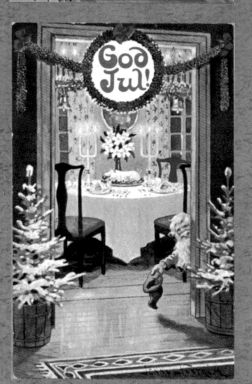

56

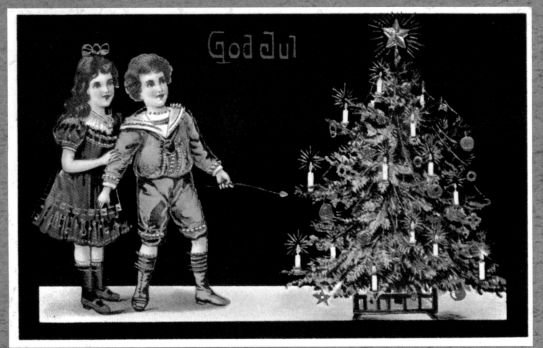

Offering by Nonbelievers   Something that comes with every Christmas celebration are the complaints about how expensive and stressful it all is. This raises the question of how a small farm in the countryside had the resources to replace its austere and strenuous daily life with one of abundance and idleness, albeit, for only a few days. Anthropologists liken the excesses of food and drink at Christmas with Pagan offerings. The offering was the prayer of primitive peoples. By having lots to eat and drink, and by being excessively benevolent toward visitors and the poor, nonbelievers hoped that the same abundance and benevolence would be afforded to them by the powers above.

The Ringing in of Christmas   At last, the peace of Christmas could be heralded by church bells or a christened tomte. This was the signal to cease any fights or petty quarrels for the duration of the holiday season. This prohibition was even stated in Sweden's ancient provincial laws. Crimes of violence during the Christmas holidays were more severely punished than those committed at other times of the year.

Anders Olsson   The artist who continued to paint Christmas cards in the traditional way for the longest time was Anders Olsson, with his characteristic decorative signature. He was as careful with details as Jenny Nyström, and this gives his numerous cards and small posters, with settings from the 1950s and 1960s, added value. Check out the fireplace! Anders Olsson's anatomical skills, so evident in his nude studies and his illustrations of "Red Indians," have been put to good use on his more muscular Santas.

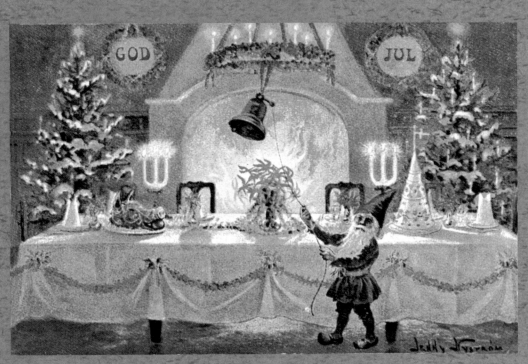

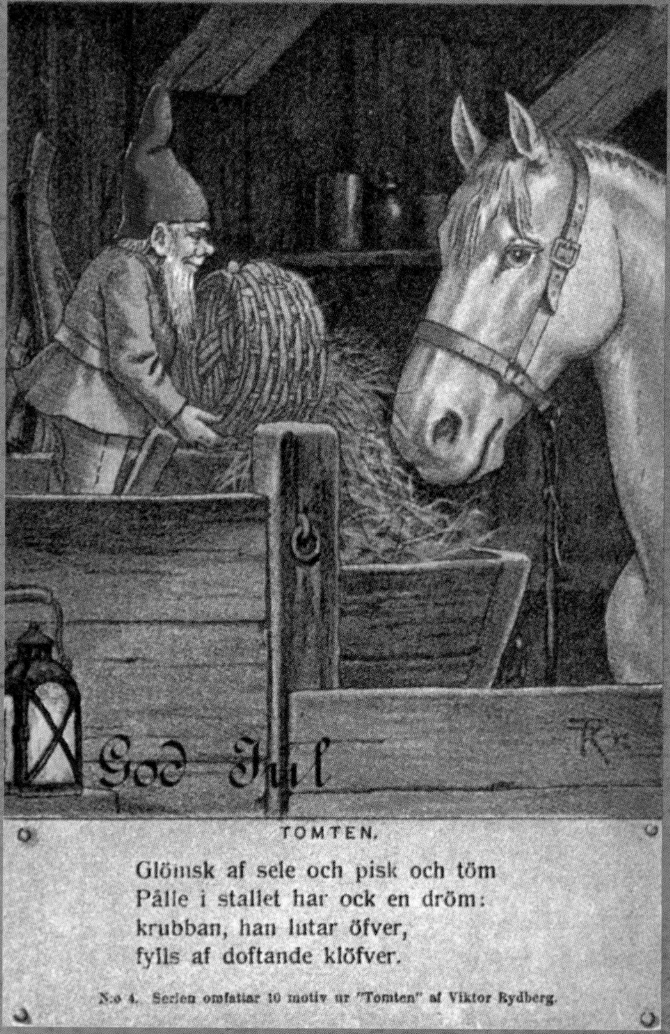

TOMTEN.

Glömsk af sele och pisk och töm
Pålle i stallet har ock en dröm:
krubban, han lutar öfver,
fylls af doftande klöfver.

N:o 4. Serien omfattar 10 motiv ur "Tomten" af Viktor Rydberg.

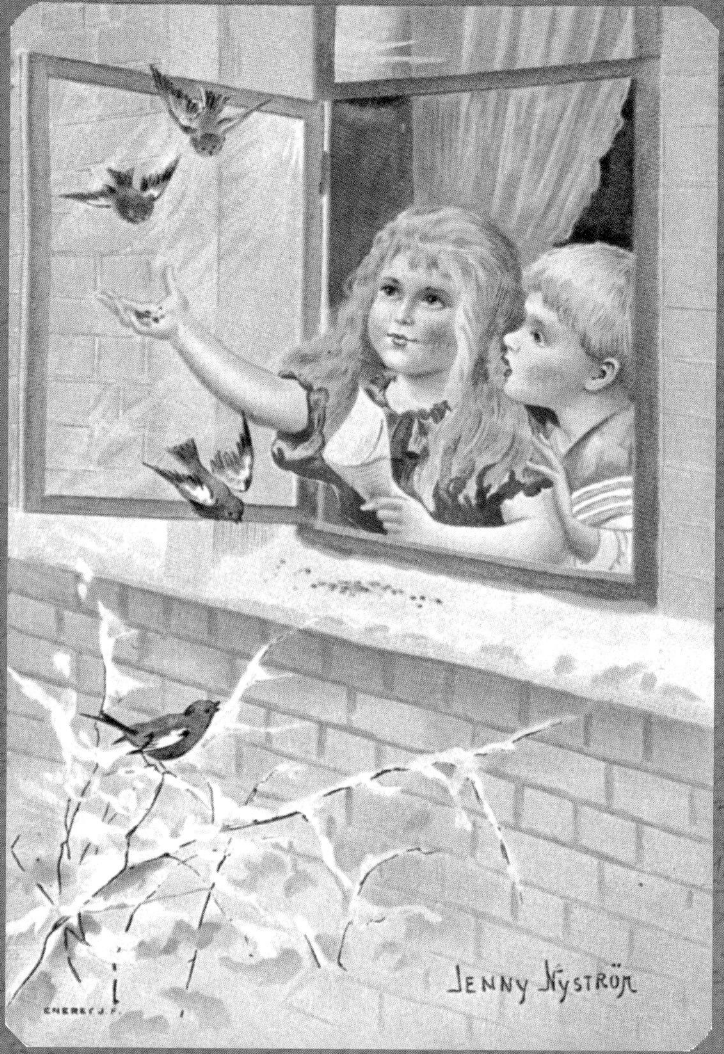

T R-n
(Torvald Rasmusson),
Wilh. Lundkvist,
Stockholm 1909.
The card was number 4
of 10 with text from the
poem *Tomten* by Viktor
Rydberg.

Jenny Nyström,
Eneret 1899.

Santa's Reward   The tomte of Swedish folklore worked hard everyday. He had the well-being of the farm in his hands, and he would take this supernatural power with him if he moved so he had to be treated well and with a lot of sensitivity. Apart from this, all he demanded in return for his goodwill, was an annual bowl of porridge. Originally, this was put out for the tomte on New Year's Eve, but after his status was raised to that of Santa, the annual reward was given on Christmas Eve. It was not only Santa who got a treat on this day; all the animals were given extra rations. The guard dogs were taken off their leashes and were even allowed to taste the Christmas porridge.

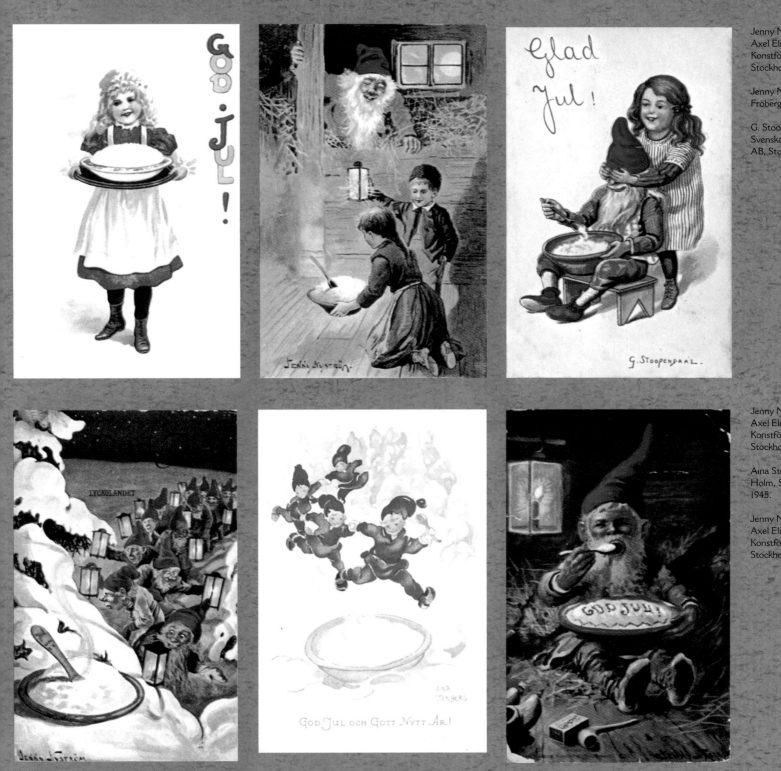

Jenny Nyström,
Axel Eliassons
Konstförlag,
Stockholm.

Jenny Nyström,
Fröbergs, Finspong.

G. Stoopendaal,
Svenska Litografiska
AB, Stockholm.

Jenny Nyström,
Axel Eliassons
Konstförlag,
Stockholm 1909.

Aina Stenberg, Eskil
Holm, Stockholm
1945.

Jenny Nyström,
Axel Eliassons
Konstförlag,
Stockholm.

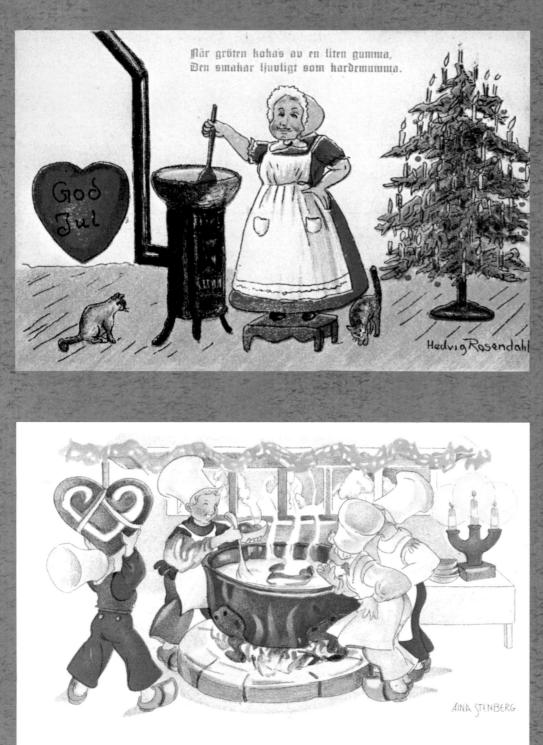

När gröten kokas av en liten gumma,
Den smakar ljuvligt som kardemumma.

God Jul

Hedvig Rosendahl

AINA STENBERG

It's Christmas Time

The Christmas Pile   On Christmas tables of old, a pile of baked goods was laid out at each setting as a form of a placement card. Sometimes names were written in sugar on the top of a wheat bun. The master of the house got the biggest Christmas pile while the rest were in proportion to each person's ranking in the household. The servants were given extra big piles as they shared them with their families. There were many symbolic values attached to the bread which was baked and shaped in accordance with ancient recipes. On top of the master's heap, there was often a loaf in the shape of a small bird with an ear of wheat in its beak and a wish for a good harvest in the coming year. The bread from the pile was not to be eaten right away and some of the baked goods were to be saved until after Christmas.

The Christmas Menu   It is simpler to list what was not on the Christmas buffet, than the other way around. The conspicuous absentee was potatoes, as they were consumed every other day of the year. The Christmas menu was dominated by the products from the newly slaughtered pig. Nothing was wasted, and the dipping of bread in the gravy, fresh ham, ribs, pigs' ears, and all the other delicacies must have been a wonderful break from a daily diet of salted and dried meat or fish. Fresh fish was not readily available at Christmas, but pickled herring and lutfisk were on the menu. During the Catholic era, only "white" food was eaten during the days leading up to the big holidays. Both the lutfisk and the Christmas porridge are remnants from that time. Porridge was eaten year-round, but rice porridge was reserved for festivities.

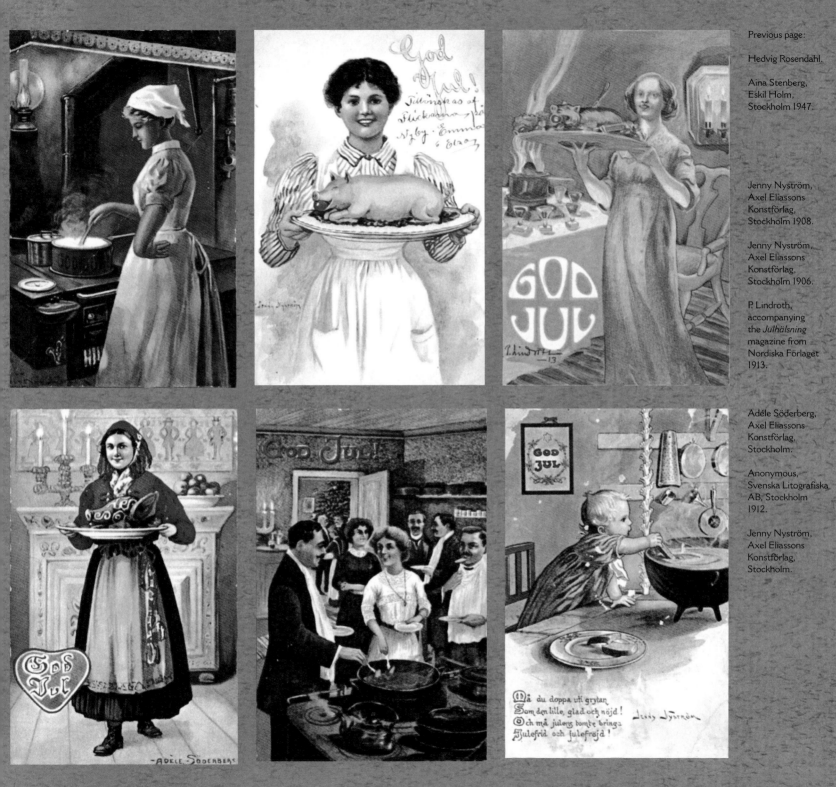

Previous page:

Hedvig Rosendahl.

Aina Stenberg,
Eskil Holm,
Stockholm 1947.

Jenny Nyström,
Axel Eliassons
Konstförlag,
Stockholm 1908.

Jenny Nyström,
Axel Eliassons
Konstförlag,
Stockholm 1906.

P. Lindroth,
accompanying
the *Julhälsning*
magazine from
Nordiska Förlaget
1913.

Adéle Söderberg,
Axel Eliassons
Konstförlag,
Stockholm.

Anonymous,
Svenska Litografiska
AB, Stockholm
1912.

Jenny Nyström,
Axel Eliassons
Konstförlag,
Stockholm.

Carl Larsson,
Förgätmigej kort
1973.

M.L. Borgh,
Axel Eliassons
Konstförlag,
Stockholm 1900–06.

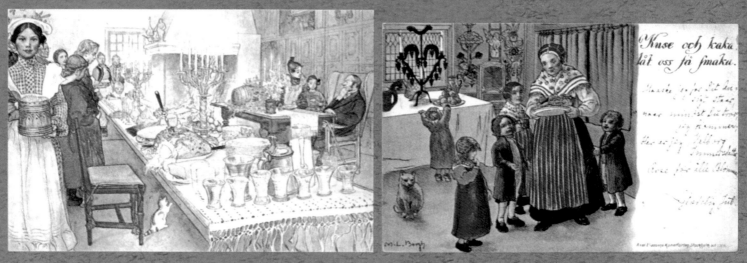

H. Larsen,
Paul Heckschers
Förlag.

Jenny Nyström,
Axel Eliassons
Konstförlag,
Stockholm 1908.

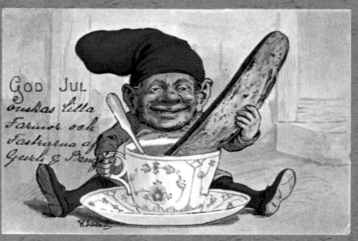

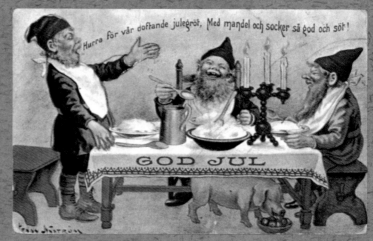

Adina Sand,
Granbergs 1917.

Jac. Edgren,
Nordisk Konst.

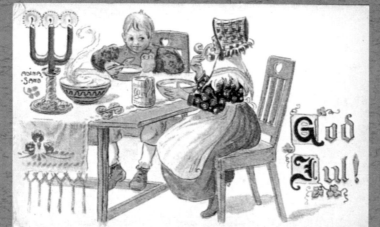

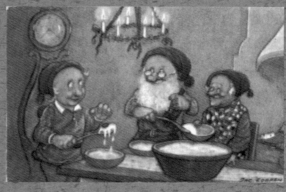

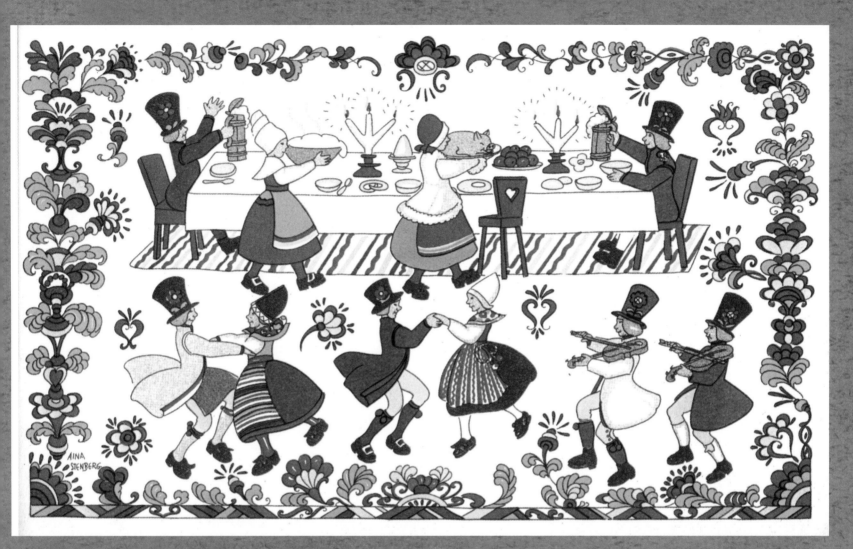

Aina Stenberg,
Eskil Holm 1947.

Angel Food The night of Christmas Eve was one of the most magical of the year. This was when an almond in the porridge could reveal who was going to get married. But before tasting the porridge, each person around the table had to recite a "porridge rhyme." All the food was left on the table because there was a belief that the recently deceased would come down for a taste on this special night. Eventually, this custom was Christianized and a little extra food was laid out as "angel food." It was not unusual for a place to be set at the table for family members who had died during the year.

Aina Stenberg,
Eskil Holm,
Stockholm.

Jenny Nyström,
Axel Eliassons
Konstförlag,
Stockholm 1910.

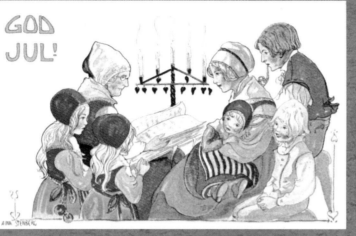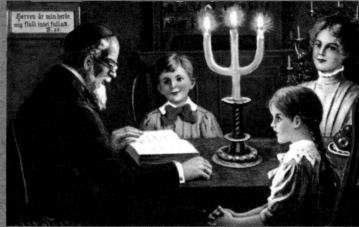

Jenny Nyström,
Axel Eliassons
Konstförlag,
Stockholm 1909.

Colored
photograph,
Åhlén & Holm,
1915.

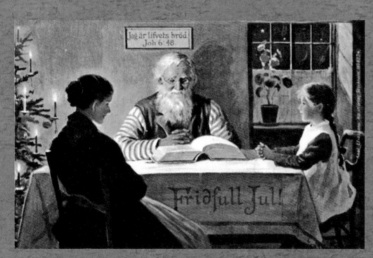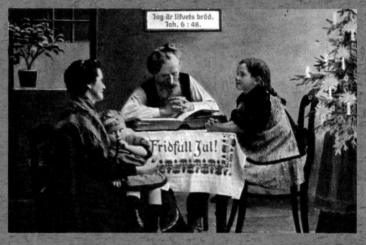

German card from
1921.

Jenny Nyström,
Nordisk Konst 1965.

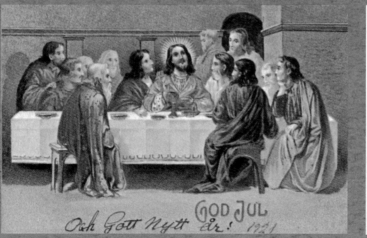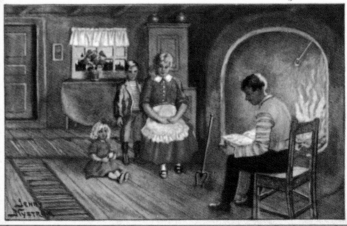

Jenny Nyström,
Axel Eliassons
Konstförlag,
Stockholm 1909.

Anonymous 1906.

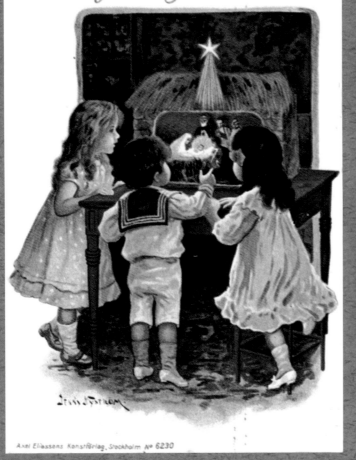

Fridfull jul !

Axel Eliassons Konstförlag, Stockholm № 6230

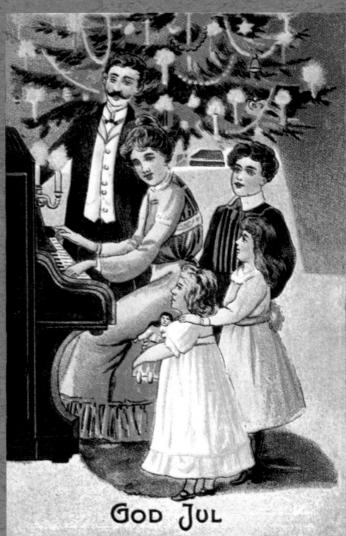

GOD JUL

Fellowship and Devotion Family and servants gathered for prayer and the singing of hymns before the more secular and merrier aspects of Christmas began in earnest. The master of the house read the gospel, and the real meaning of Christmas was proclaimed. Older Christmas cards very often have a religious theme, and about a quarter of cards today still come with a religious message. Apart from scenes of the family gathered around the bible and motifs inspired by the Last Supper, there are cards with Jesus in the crib, the expedition to the Christmas Day morning church service, landscapes with churches, a ringing church bell, and angels. When a family gathering is depicted on a card, it most often comes with all the upper middle class trimmings. Just as in contemporary family photographs, the handsome parents and well-behaved children are captured in stiff poses.

Anonymous,
Alex. Vincent's
Kunstforlag,
Eneberettiget.

C. Hedelin's
"Skånsk jul,"
Tullbergs
Konsindustri AB
1895.

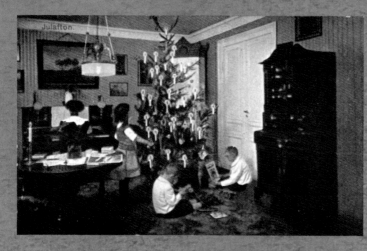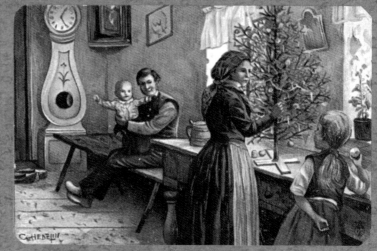

Photo by Gerda
Söderlund,
Axel Eliassons
Konstförlag,
Stockholm 1910.

Gold-embossed
card, PBF, 1911.

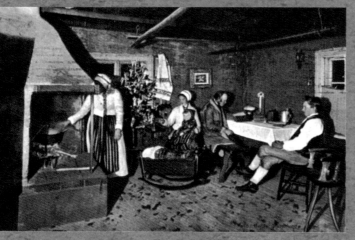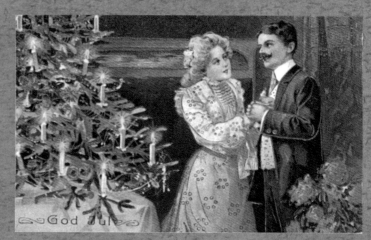

Hildur Söderberg,
1917.

Colored
photograph.

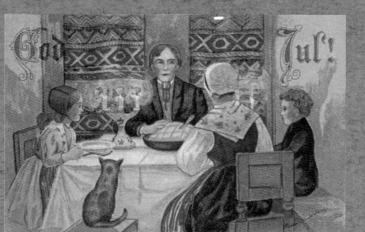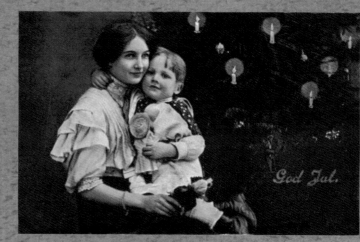

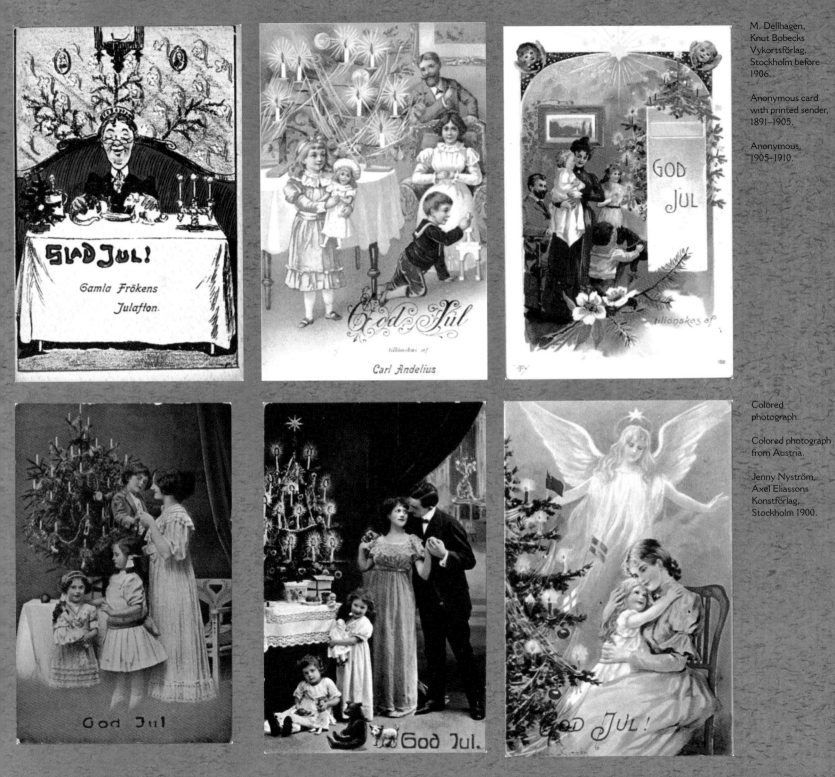

M. Dellhagen,
Knut Bobecks
Vykortsförlag,
Stockholm before
1906.

Anonymous card
with printed sender,
1891–1905.

Anonymous,
1905–1910.

Colored
photograph.

Colored photograph
from Austria.

Jenny Nyström,
Axel Eliassons
Konstförlag,
Stockholm 1900.

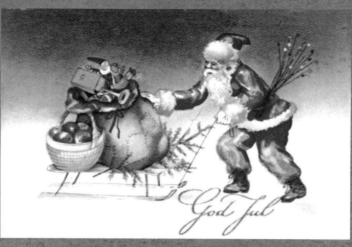

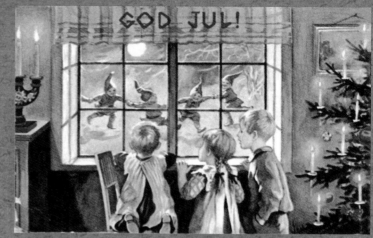

Hannes Petersen,
HWB, 1930.

Jenny Nyström,
Axel Eliassons
Konstförlag,
Stockholm 1912.

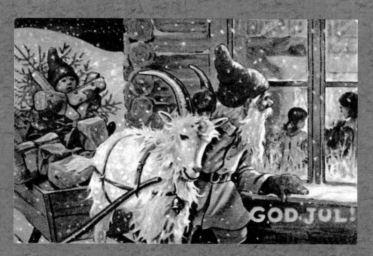

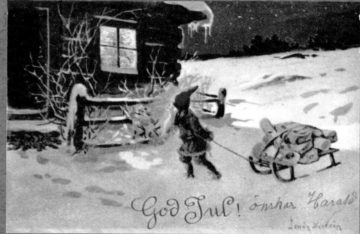

Jenny Nyström,
Axel Eliassons
Konstförlag,
Stockholm 1916.

Jenny Nyström,
Axel Eliassons
Konstförlag,
Stockholm 1906.

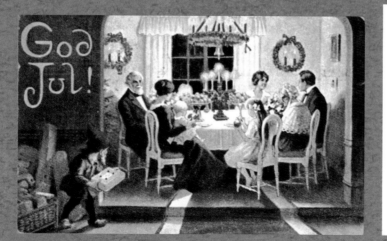

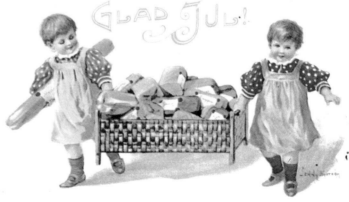

Jenny Nyström,
Axel Eliassons
Konstförlag,
Stockholm.

Jenny Nyström,
Axel Eliassons
Konstförlag,
Stockholm 1906.

Jenny Nyström,
Axel Eliassons
Konstförlag,
Stockholm 1904
(reproduction of
older motif).

Jenny Nyström,
Axel Eliassons
Konstförlag,
Stockholm 1915.

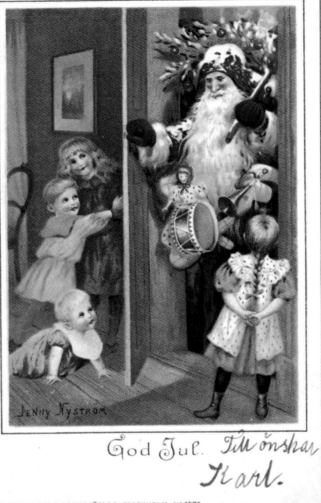

God Jul. Till önskar
Karl.

AXEL ELIASSONS KONSTFÖRLAG STOCKHOLM. Nº 1571.

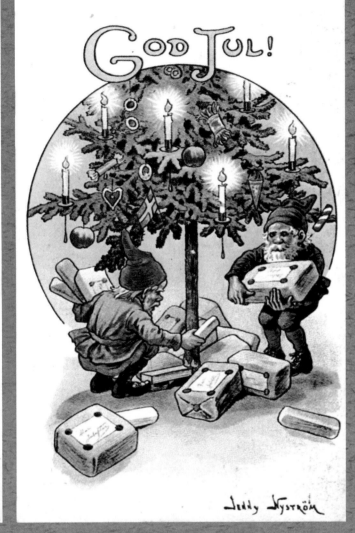

GOD JUL!

Santa Arrives At last he is here, the long-awaited Santa. And in Sweden, he comes to the house in person. He does not look much like he does in the pictures, but he is here. It has been a full year of toil for all the small "nissar" or gnomes who make the toys and other gifts in the Christmas gift factory at the North Pole or in Lappland. The same toys are strangely enough available in the stores downtown. Mum and Dad have apparently bought the gifts in the store but Santa helps to distribute them. And he comes from far away to do that. As usual, Dad misses Santa's visit as he is away on a last-minute errand. And Santa is always in a hurry as he has to make it to so many children's homes. He is warmly thanked as he waves goodbye and leaves with his empty sack. Eventually Dad returns and is so disappointed that he once again missed Santa's visit.

Anonymous, EAS
1910.

Hand-painted card
from the Stockholm
Postal Museum
collection, 1917.

Jenny Nyström,
Axel Eliassons
Konstförlag,
Stockholm 1917.

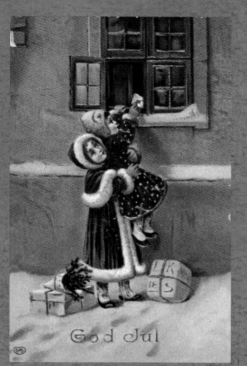

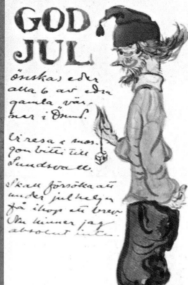

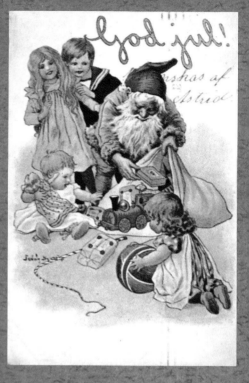

Anonymous, EAS.

Jenny Nyström,
portrait of son Curt,
1906–1908.

Jenny Nyström,
Axel Eliassons
Konstförlag,
Stockholm.

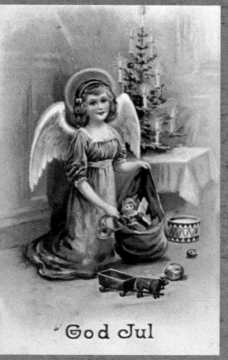

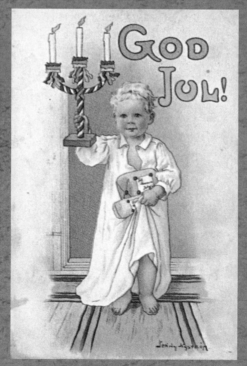

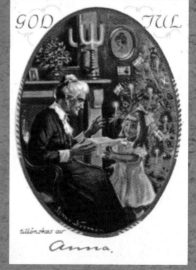

70

E. Blomberg,
Jolin & Wilkenson
Konstförlag, Göteborg 1918.

Anonymous, Axel Eliassons
Konstförlag, Stockholm 1903.

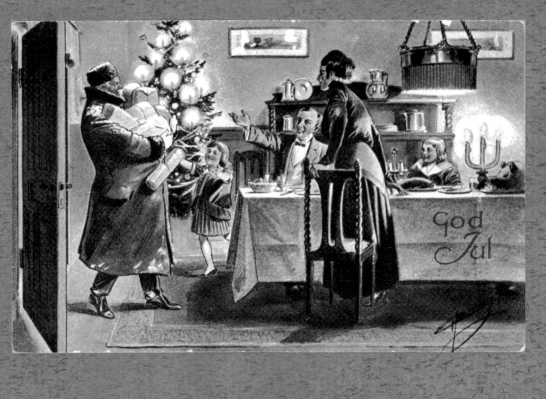

The Christmas Gift   Gift giving at Christmas has a very modest beginning. It may all have started with the St. Nicholas gift on December 6. Or it could have been the New Year's gift that was so popular at one time but has now completely disappeared. Or it might have started with the tasty treats that servants and others received at Christmas. But the origin could just as well have been the little humorous rhyme or funny object that was given anonymously with a bit of gamesmanship. The idea was to knock on someone's door on Christmas Eve or on one of the following days, quickly throw in the so-called gift on the floor, and make a quick getaway. The recipients, pursuing the giver, more often than not in vain, would in turn try and get rid of the embarrassing gift in the same way so as not to be the final butt of the joke. In Swedish, the Christmas gift is called *julklapp* which literally translates into the "Christmas pat" on the door.

The Christmas Goat   One of the most popular dress-up clothes for men in the olden days was to wear the fur coat inside out, that is with the fur lining on the outside. With horns and a beard added and a special gait to boot, you had a perfect goat. This is how the little devil, who accompanied St. Nicholas on his gift-giving expeditions, was dressed. Before Santa came around toward the end of the 19th century, the goat had taken on the important role of the distributor of gifts in Sweden. Today the goat, made of straw, has been relegated to a popular Christmas decoration in all Swedish homes. There have historically been attempts to have Little Jesus or the angels bring the gifts but Santa seems to have emerged as the undisputed victor in this competition.

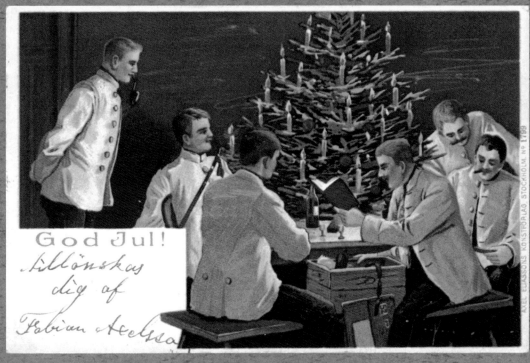

God Jul!
Tillönskas
dig af
Fabian Axelssa

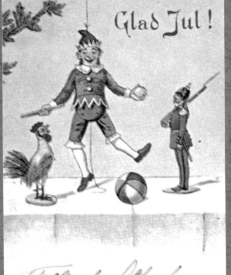

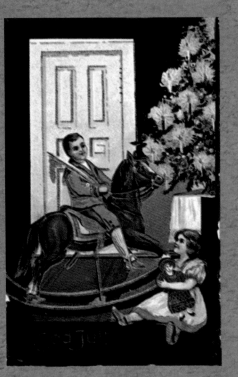

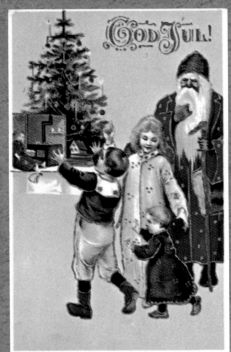

T R-n
(Torvald
Rasmussen),
Eskilstuna
Fotografiska
Magasin, Eskilstuna
1904.

Anonymous, 1912.

Anonymous, SB,
1914.

Anonymous
German card, 1909.

Robert Högfeldt,
1957.

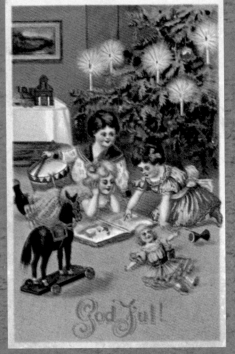

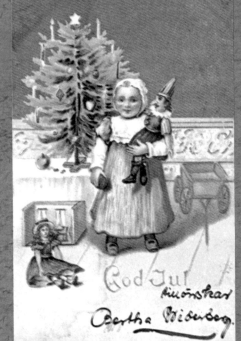

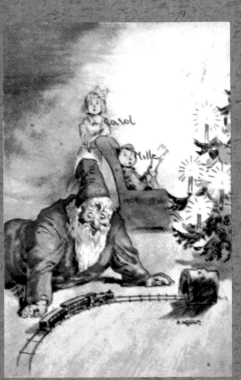

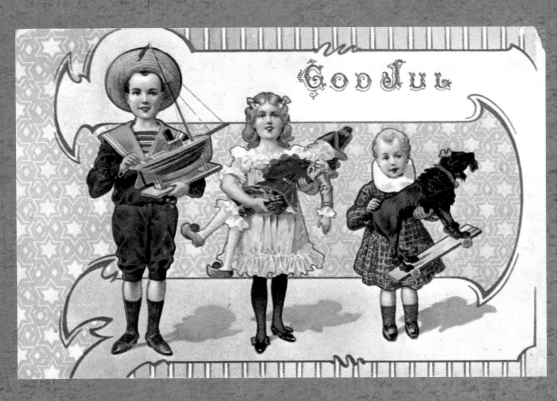

Toys The earliest toys given as Christmas gifts were wooden figures and dolls made out of straw. They were very primitive compared to the toys that were beginning to be produced in factories. The pretty playthings on the Christmas cards were the domain of privileged children. For others these were the subject of dreams that they could closely study on the cards they received. There were dolls with the most precious little porcelain faces and exquisite wardrobes. After 1870, there were also ingenious mechanical toys produced in Germany. Tin soldiers and swords were some of the many popular military toys. But this was also a time when just a pen and paper would have been very gratefully received.

Robert Högfeldt Then as now, toys were chosen by the parents. So a father dressed up in a Santa suit playing with the mechanical train, while the children look on, is probably quite a true-to-life image. Dutch-born Robert Högfeldt was skilled at coming up with hilarious settings for his small and plump jovial figures. His lithographic posters are now being rediscovered just like a lot of other popular art that did not fit into the criteria of serious art of the past.

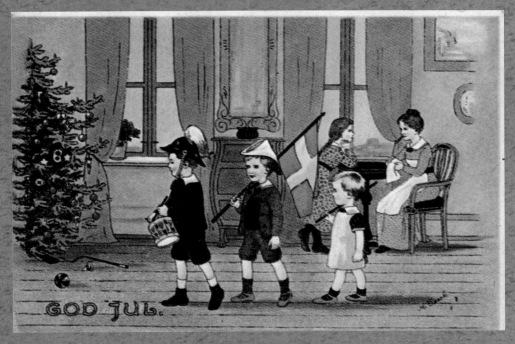

Opposite page:

The signature H.B., A.V., Copenhagen 1904.

Amalia Lindgrens "Dance in the Dalecarlian cottage," H.L.J., Stockholm 1902.

Semmy Nyström, Granbergs 1915.

Anonymous, AB Oscar E. Kulls Grafiska Konst-Anstalt, Malmö.

G. Stoopendaal, Sv. Litografiska AB, 1914.

Jenny Nyström, Axel Eliassons Konstförlag, Stockholm 1908.

The signature T.N., G.K.A. 1904.

G. Stoopendaal, Åhlén & Holm, 1900.

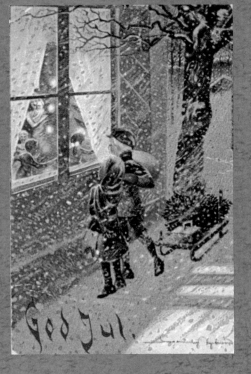

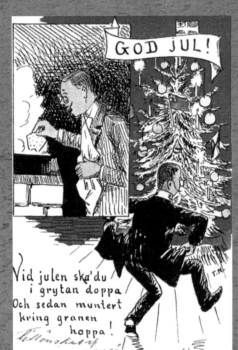

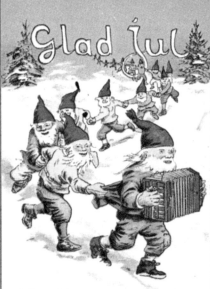

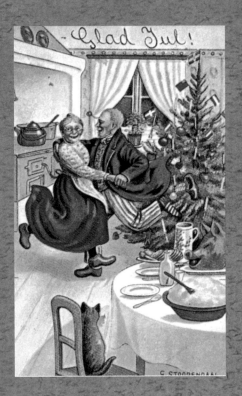

The Fox Scuttles Over the Ice

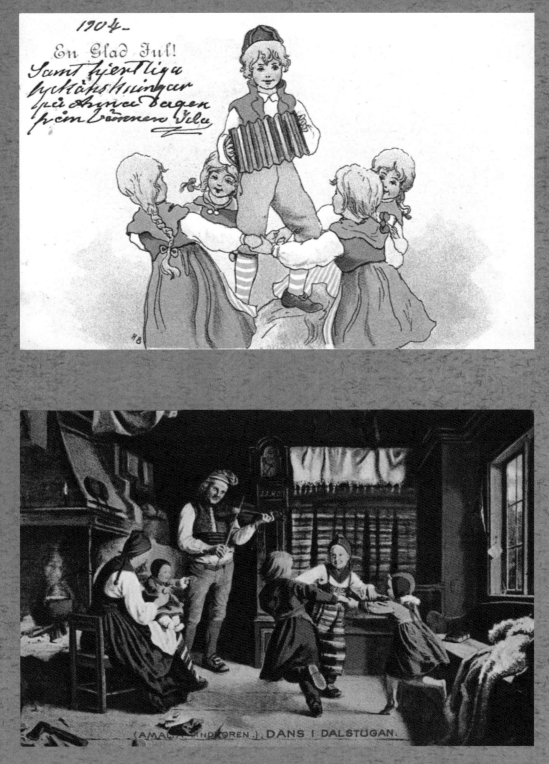

1904—
En Glad Jul!

Dancing Around the Christmas Tree
Dancing around the Christmas tree is obviously a tradition dating back not longer than the Christmas tree itself. However, even before there was a tree, there was always dancing and games after the sumptuous Christmas meal. Servants socialized with their masters on an equal footing during the democratic Christmas holiday. The wooden clogs stayed on even indoors as the carpets had been replaced by straw. It was fun to romp around on this comfortable flooring. Men excelled at different games of strength while the whole family joined in for games like *Blind Man's Buff* and the Swedish dance games Skära, Skära Havre and The Fox Scuttles over the Ice, which are mentioned as early as the 17th and 18th centuries. Most homes had very little space, so most of the serious dancing took place at the communal parties or "playhouses" as they were also called. This is where youth, old enough to have been confirmed, met to dance, play, and consume all the food and drink that they had collected after a little begging from the adults.

Georg Stoopendaal   The happy couple dancing in the kitchen, as well as the Santas' ring dance were produced by Georg Stoopendaal. His Christmas cards are full of novel ideas. He was the brother-in-law of Jenny Nyström and had received much of his training from her. She recommended him when she did not have time herself for all the commissions she received, but was not happy when she had to field complaints about his delays and carelessness. Georg Stoopendaal emigrated to the United States and even had a stint as a war correspondent in Cuba before he returned to Sweden. There were many artists in the Stoopendaal family including Jenny Nyström's husband, Daniel Stoopendaal, who sometimes helped her with her painting.

(AMALIA LINDGREN.) DANS I DALSTUGAN.

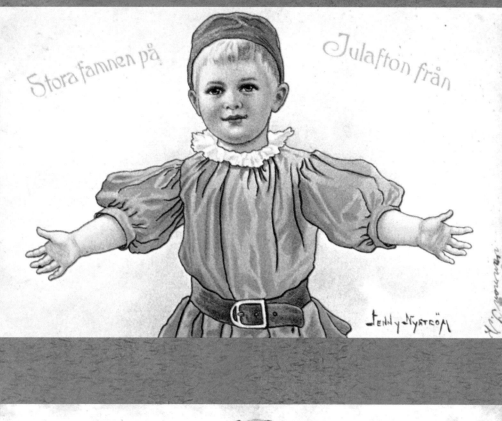

Hugs and Kisses

The Mistletoe   The mistletoe has always had an aura of being somewhat magical. At Christmas it has been used, together with holly, as a form of protection on or above doors. In Sweden, where there is little holly, lingonberry twigs with strong leaves and red berries are the norm. The kissing under the mistletoe started in England and Swedes were quick to adopt the custom. But kisses could also be used as prizes in games. Hence, it is not surprising that they also made their way into Christmas cards.

Valentine Cards   Quite a few of the kisses on cards have nothing whatsoever to do with Christmas. These cards are rather Valentine cards gone haywire. Celebrated on February 14, the St. Valentine celebration started in the Anglo-Saxon countries where anonymous expressions of love to somebody long admired from afar were sent on this day. The wishful thinking found expression in motifs of hugs and kisses. Swedish card producers added Christmas or Easter wishes to these motifs, as a St. Valentine celebration had not yet made it to Sweden. This gave rise to the Easter kiss and a whole new range of Christmas motifs.

Swedish Christmas Card Publishers   It was Jenny Nyström who, while studying abroad, saw Christmas cards and alerted the venerable Bonnier publishing house about them. "They are very much in fashion abroad, and I think they would do well at home, where so much shabbiness of this kind is bought by the public," she argued. Bonniers was not interested, so Jenny

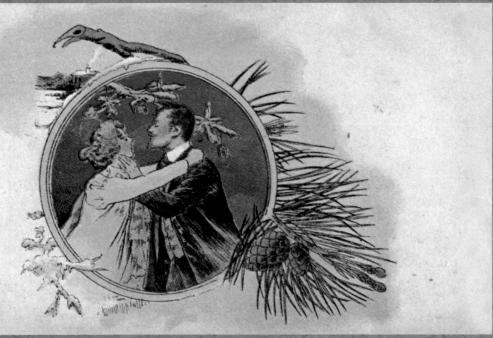

Nyström made her first designs for Eskil Holm in Stockholm and John Fröberg in Finspong. She had already painted a few originals for Wards in London, one of the largest card producers in Europe at the time. Eventually Axel Eliassons Konstförlag in Stockholm became the exclusive producer of Jenny Nyström cards and sells them to this day. Axel Eliasson had studied the very skilled German card producers before he, as a 22-year-old, set up his own publishing business. From a modest beginning in 1891, with a couple of motifs from Stockholm and Gothenburg, Axel Eliassons Konstförlag is today the only one of the many Swedish postcard producers with an unbroken tradition. Other pioneers were Tullbergs, Granbergs, and many others represented in this book.

The Widening of the Christmas Greeting
Holiday cards eventually developed into a real industry. In the 1950s, there was a reaction against the impersonal and formal habit of sending Christmas cards, but ironically this resulted in even more cards. Nineteen ninety-six was a top year for Christmas cards in Sweden with 62 million mailed. Since then there has been a steady drop with electronic greetings steadily gaining new ground. Many businesses have also replaced cards with diaries, calendars, or gift baskets. In the U.S., Christmas is still the biggest season for cards, with about 1.9 billion mailed each year.

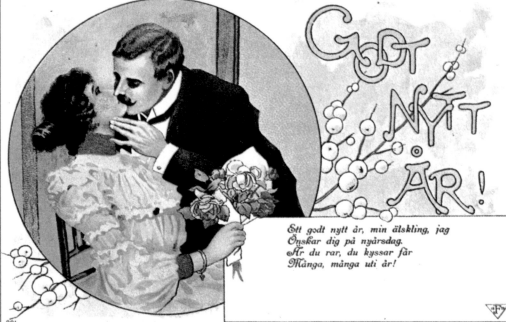

281

Ett godt nytt år, min älskling, jag
Önskar dig på nyårsdag.
Är du rar, du kyssar får
Många, många uti år!

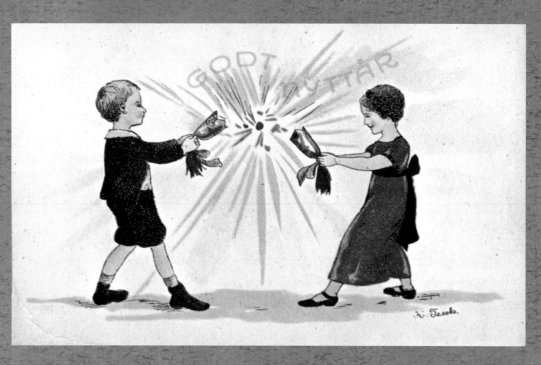

H. Teschs, E.F.P.

Jenny Nyström,
without any
publisher's name,
1906.

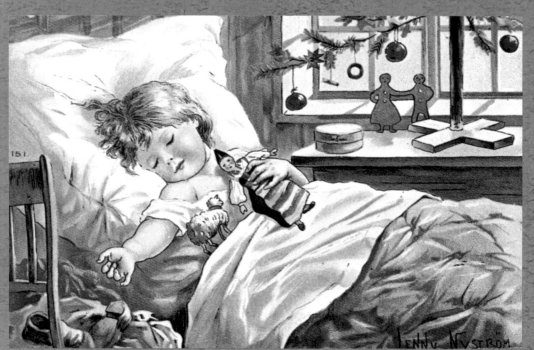

Magical Night   When the last of the sparklers had died down and the last of the crackers silenced, it was bedtime for the little ones. In the olden days the family would sometimes bed down in the straw on the floor on this magical night, to leave the proper beds for the spirits of any dead relatives. The husband was not allowed to sleep next to his wife on this night. Candles were left to burn for the spirits and perhaps plain and simply because it felt good with some light on a dark night such as this. What was left of the candles in the morning was collected and used as medication during the coming year. Candle wax was good to have around to soothe a child's sore bum or when the cow's teats needed smoothing. The supernatural powers had complete control over the magical Christmas night. Hence, it was best to paint the sign of the cross on each door to stop evil powers from entering the house. Before going to bed, all tools had to be brought indoors because otherwise they would be destroyed by the next morning.

Predicting the Future   Ashes from the Christmas night fire, which were believed to have magical powers, were spread across the fields. It was not uncommon to rub some ashes on farm animals to prevent them from getting any diseases during the year. But before any ashes were collected, they had to be closely examined because they contained all kinds of valuable information about the coming year. If there were, for example, tracks in the ashes in the direction of the room, there would be an addition to the family. If the tracks were directed outward, there would be a death in the coming year. There were other ways to look into the future on Christmas night—at least for those who dared. The recommended way was the "year walk." It called for fasting on Christmas Eve (the very idea!) and then without uttering a single word, walking past seven churches and looking in through their keyholes. Everything that was observed on the walk home from the last church would have a significance for the coming year. That is, if it was interpreted correctly. The worst that could happen would be an encounter with the terrible, folkloristic *gloson* which was some kind of evil, Christmas pig. Its only function in life was to run in between the legs of a person and split him or her in two with its knife-sharp back.

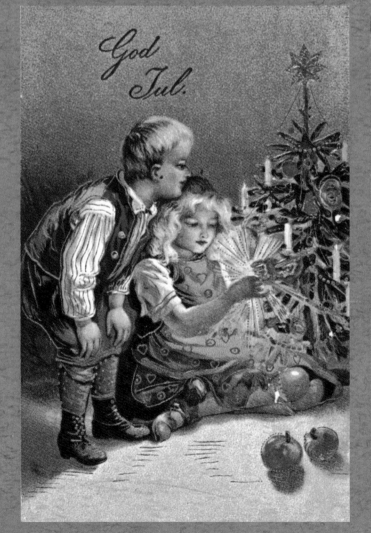

Anonymous, P.B.F.

Jenny Nyström's:
"John Blund",
Axel Eliassons
Konstförlag during
the 19th century.

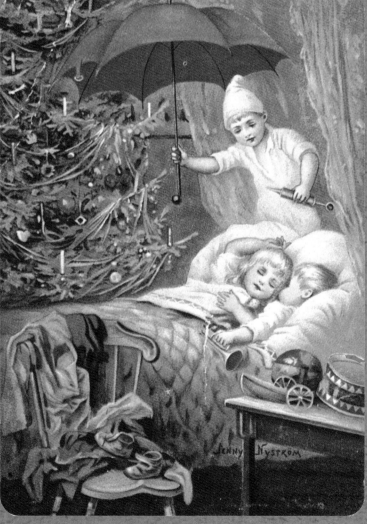

Aina Stenberg,
Eskil Holm,
Stockholm 1947.

Aina Stenberg,
Eski Holm,
Stockholm 1938.

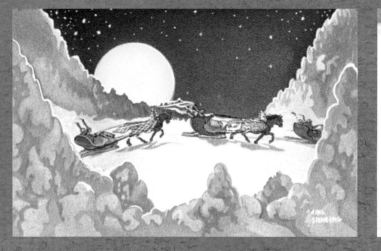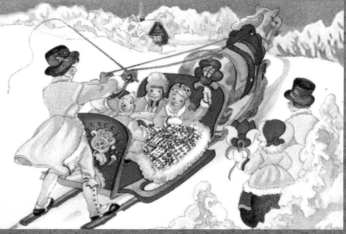

Curt Nyström
Stoopendaal,
Axel Eliassons
Konstförlag,
Stockholm.

Aina Stenberg,
Eskil Holm,
Stockholm 1939
(73, 76).

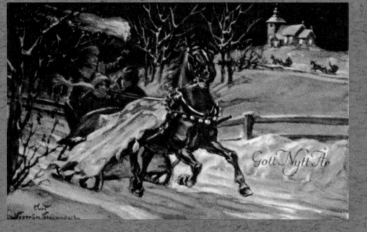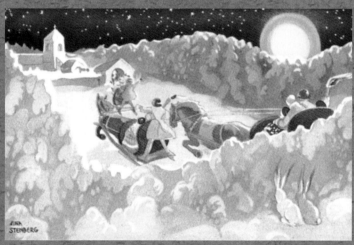

Aina Stenberg,
Eskil Holm,
Stockholm 1934.

Aina Stenberg,
Eskil Holm,
Stockholm 1945.

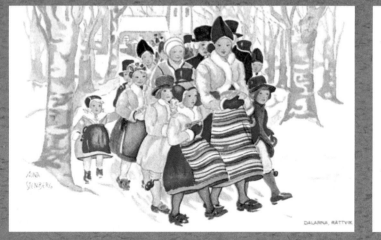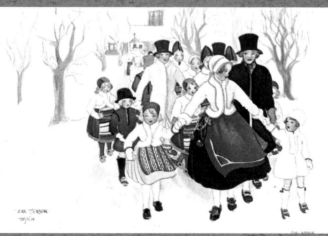

Jenny Nyström,
Axel Eliassons
Konstförlag,
Stockholm.

Anonymous
1905–1910.

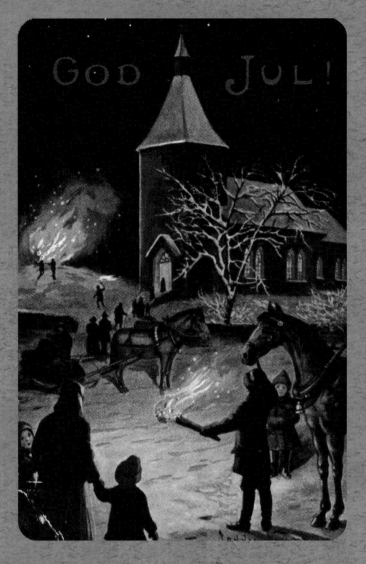

GOD JUL!

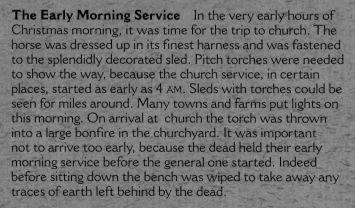

When Christmas Morning Glistens

The Early Morning Service   In the very early hours of Christmas morning, it was time for the trip to church. The horse was dressed up in its finest harness and was fastened to the splendidly decorated sled. Pitch torches were needed to show the way, because the church service, in certain places, started as early as 4 AM. Sleds with torches could be seen for miles around. Many towns and farms put lights on this morning. On arrival at church the torch was thrown into a large bonfire in the churchyard. It was important not to arrive too early, because the dead held their early morning service before the general one started. Indeed before sitting down the bench was wiped to take away any traces of earth left behind by the dead.

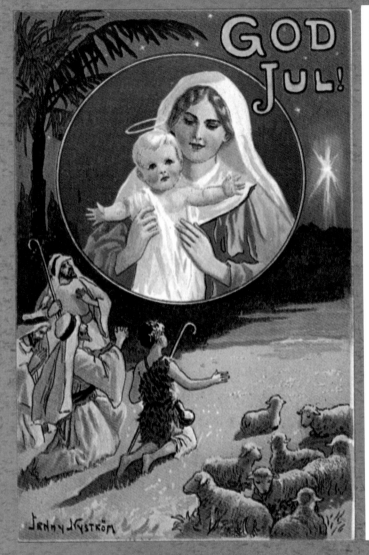

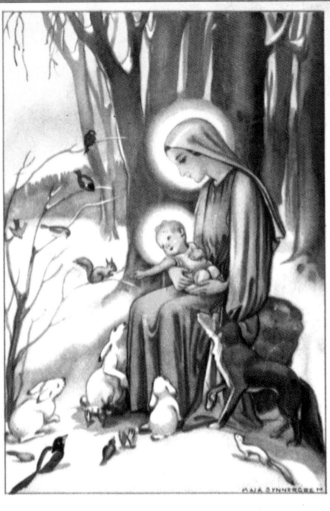

Jenny Nyström,
Axel Eliassons
Konstförlag,
Stockholm 1906.

Maja Synnergren
1941.

The Race   With the early morning service done with, it was time for a race. The belief was that the family that reached home first would also be the first to get the harvest in. To better the odds, farm hands were known to sneak out during the sermon and switch the harnesses of their competitors to cause a bit of confusion, and in that way, get a head start. Apart from this, the Christmas card motifs of the morning service project a feeling of peace. There are motifs where the Santas seemed to have made it to the church service. Jenny Nyström has painted one tomte helping to put up the hymn numbers inside, but her six Santas sitting outside the church, with a cauldron of *glögg*, look reassuringly heathen.

Adéle Söderberg,
Axel Eliassons
Konstförlag,
Stockholm 1912.

Jenny Nyström,
Axel Eliassons
Konstförlag,
Stockholm 1908.

Unsigned Jenny
Nyström card,
printed in Germany
in 1912.

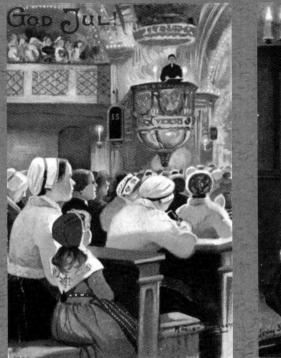 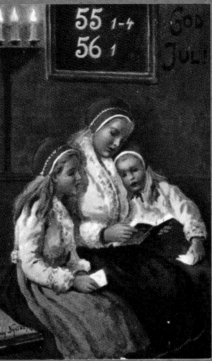 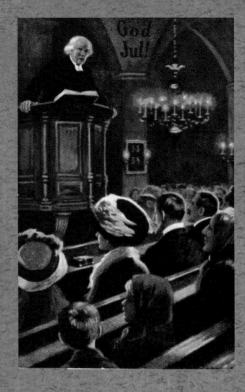

Anonymous, A.V.,
Copenhagen 1903.

Photography,
R&K, 1913.

Jenny Nyström,
Axel Eliassons
Konstförlag,
Stockholm (of a
card first published
in 1899).

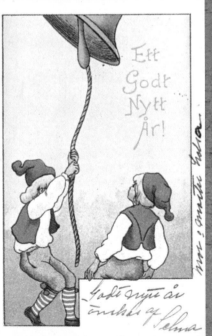 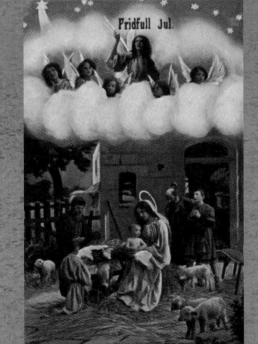 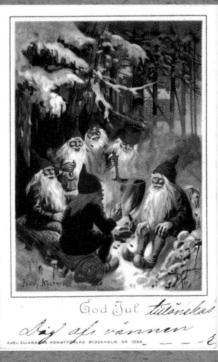

Opposite page:

C. Hall,
Eskil Holm,
Stockholm 1903.

Aina Stenberg,
Eskil Holm,
Stockholm 1947.

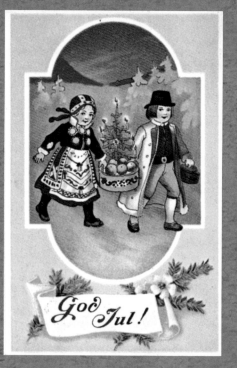

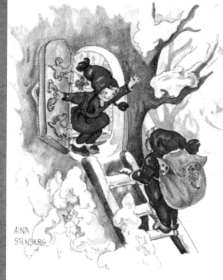

Jenny Nyström,
import without
name of producer.

Jenny Nyström,
Axel Eliassons
Konstförlag,
Stockholm 1912.

Anonymous, Joh.
Ol. Andreens
Konstförlag,
Göteborg 1905.

Anonymous.

Alna Stenberg,
Eskil Holm,
Stockholm 1950
(reprinted 1947,
1969, 1976).

Jenny Nyström,
John Fröberg,
Finspong.

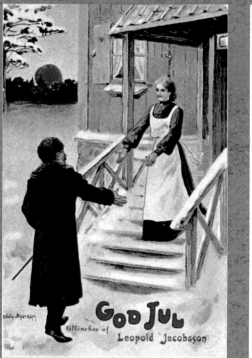

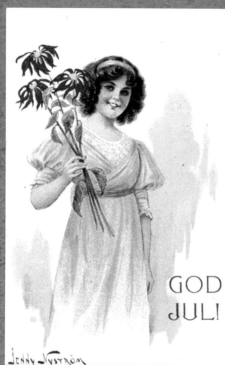

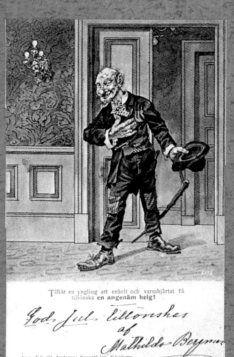

Be Greeted Both Master and Mistress

A Day of Rest Christmas Day was a day to rest at home after the hectic Christmas Eve and the early morning church service. No work was allowed on this day. Instead, Dad relaxed with Christmas magazines, like *Jultomten*, that all had a Santa taking the pride of place in their mastheads, while the children were busy with their gifts and the *Tomtepåsen* magazine full of games. The mother was in all likelihood busy in the kitchen, as usual, but hopefully she took a few breaks and indulged in the magazines *Christmas Mood* and *Mother's Christmas Letter*. No visits were allowed on Christmas Day, but the home was likely to be full anyway with extended family visiting. Anyone and everyone who could, spent the holiday with family and this included distant relatives as well as close friends.

Staffan's Ride On Boxing Day, it was once again time to get up early. The animals had not been taken care of on Christmas Day so there was lots to do. As their first task, farmhands rode out to exercise the horses that had been stabled for a long time. The horses were watered down in a north-flowing stream or spring for the sake of the magical power. Then the "Staffan's ride" would continue to the neighboring farms with the hope of getting a shot of aquavit and something good to eat. "Staffan Was a Stable Boy" was sung with a couple of improvised verses indicating what food and drink would hit the spot. If there was no hospitality forthcoming, the gang of riders would sometimes ride right into the house and help themselves.

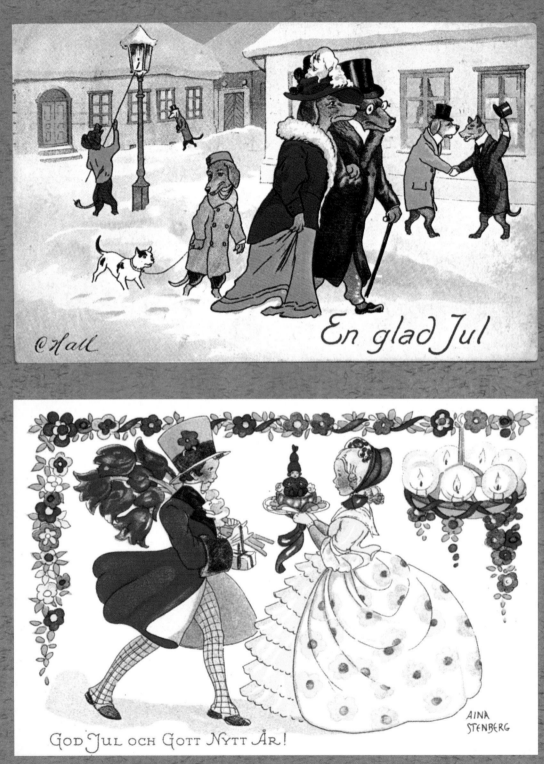

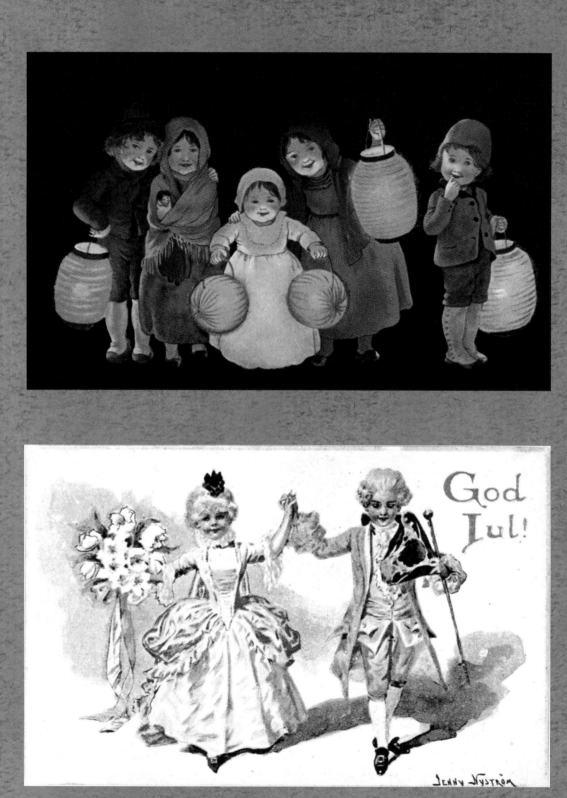

Anonymous
(who has also drawn
Asian-looking
Santas) 1916.

Jenny Nyström,
Axel Eliassons
Konstförlag,
Stockholm 1915.

God Jul!

JENNY NYSTRÖM

Play House It was not necessary to have a horse to ingratiate oneself with the neighboring farms. Maids and farmhands would also dress up and visit the farms, singing "Good Evening ye Master and Wife," for some eating and drinking. They would also collect food and drink for the communal dances to be held. Some dressed up as "star boys," but mostly the idea was to be unrecognizable. Sometimes the group would be accompanied by a Christmas goat in the form of one or more people hidden under a fur, maneuvering a ram's head with horns. Aquavit could be poured directly into the mouth of some of the more advanced goats, where the precious liquid was collected in a hidden bottle contraption.

Entertainment In the olden days, people knew so many more games than we do today. There was never a dull moment. Charades, where one person acted out an old saying without uttering a word while the others tried to guess what it was, could go on for hours on end. There were so many games that were played with just fingers that to younger children looked like plain magic. Finger dexterity also developed into full shadow plays that were especially popular in the towns. Some performers were so talented that their acts developed into theatre productions. Cinemas did brisk business long before Donald Duck's Christmas Parade became a must for families with children in the 1950s.

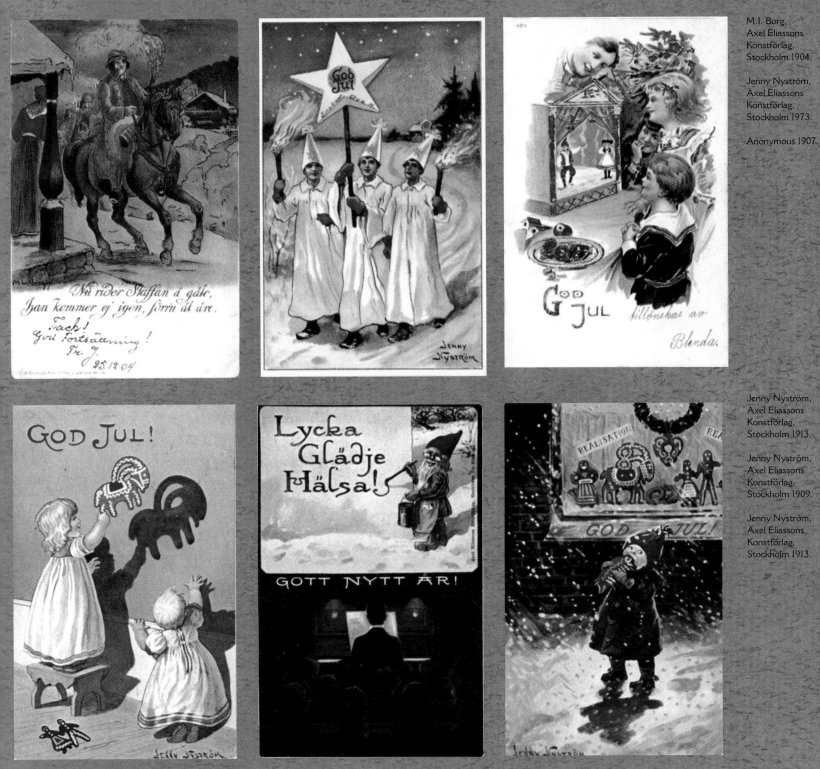

M.I. Borg,
Axel Eliassons
Konstförlag,
Stockholm 1904.

Jenny Nyström,
Axel Eliassons
Konstförlag,
Stockholm 1973.

Anonymous 1907.

Jenny Nyström,
Axel Eliassons
Konstförlag,
Stockholm 1913.

Jenny Nyström,
Axel Eliassons
Konstförlag,
Stockholm 1909.

Jenny Nyström,
Axel Eliassons
Konstförlag,
Stockholm 1913.

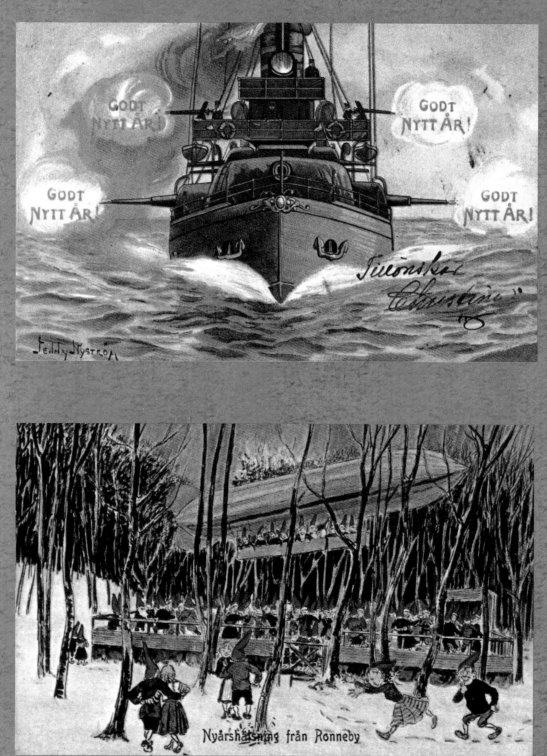

Nyårshälsning från Ronneby

Happy New Year!

Symbols of Happiness   The funniest New Year's cards are the ones with rose-colored dreams of the future. There is a veritable inflation in lucky symbols like galoshes, horseshoes, chimney sweepers, champagne, four-leaf clovers, and, above all, money. During the time of crisis, Jenny Nyström's little Santa even arrives with special lucky rationing cards, that guarantee happiness during the worst of circumstances. The biggest symbols of happiness, however, are the children that appear on so many of the cards. There are cards where Santa delivers both the newly born and the crib in the new year. On the other hand, bears on cards came with outstanding bills. But these two bears look so jovial that they could hardly be taking the debt all too seriously.

New Year's Cards   Until 1915 in Sweden, New Year's cards were far more popular than Christmas cards. Today, the rare New Year's card is probably sent by someone in reciprocation for a Christmas card received. Generally, New Year's cards have been a bit more elegant and proper and sent to people with whom the relationship is more of a formal one. New Year's cards contained wishes and invocations for the future. Santa and the bliss he represented lived on in New Year's cards. This is not so strange as Santa, in his role as caretaker of the property, had a presence throughout the year. He was also the ruler of a Land of Happiness that is every person's dream.

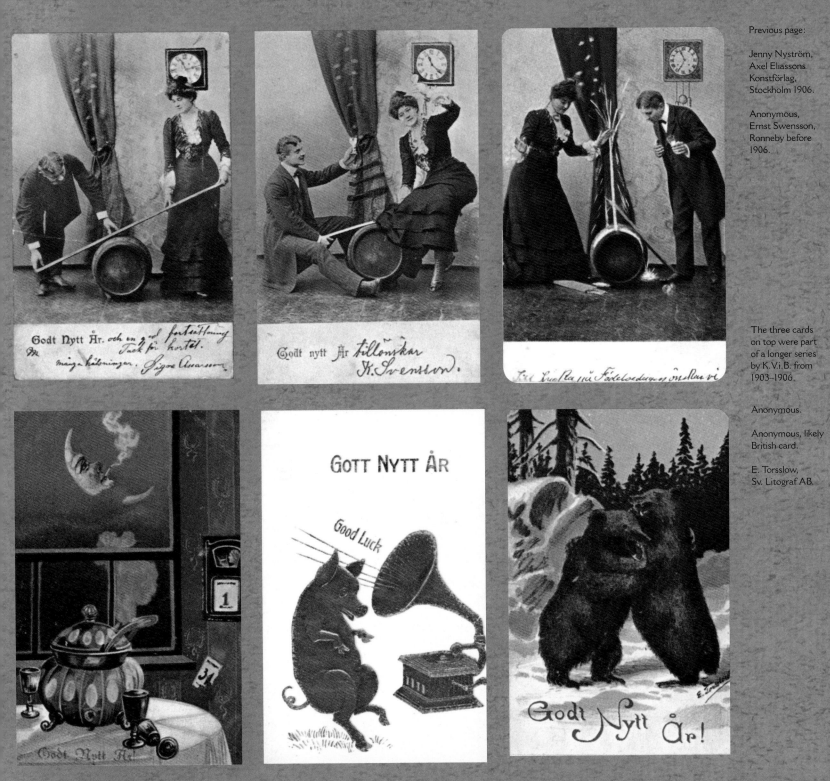

Previous page:

Jenny Nyström,
Axel Eliassons
Konstförlag,
Stockholm 1906.

Anonymous,
Ernst Swensson,
Ronneby before
1906.

The three cards
on top were part
of a longer series
by K.V.i.B. from
1903–1906.

Anonymous.

Anonymous, likely
British card.

E. Torsslow,
Sv. Litograf AB.

Godt Nytt År. och en god fortsättning. Tack för hortet. många hälsningar. Signe Arsensson.

Godt nytt År tillönskar K. Svensson.

Det lycka nu Fädelsedagen önskar vi

GOTT NYTT ÅR

Good Luck

Godt Nytt År!

Jenny Nyström,
Axel Eliassons
Konstförlag,
Stockholm 1907.

Anonymous, John
Fröberg, 1904.

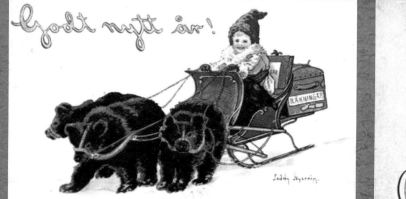

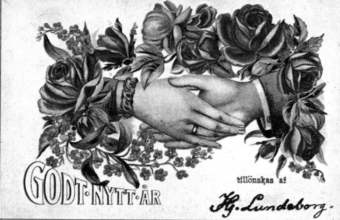

Jenny Nyström,
Axel Eliassons
Konstförlag,
Stockholm 1910.

Jenny Nyström,
Axel Eliassons
Konstförlag,
Stockholm 1910.

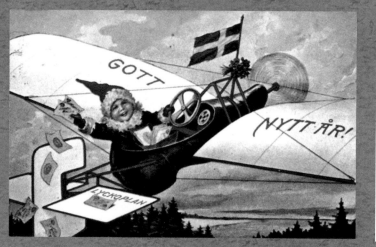

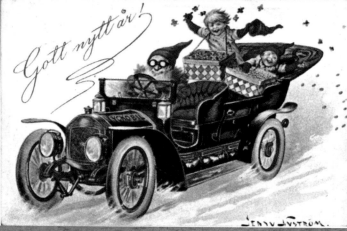

Anonymous
German card from
WB & Co.

Aina Stenberg,
Eskil Holm,
Stockholm 1917.

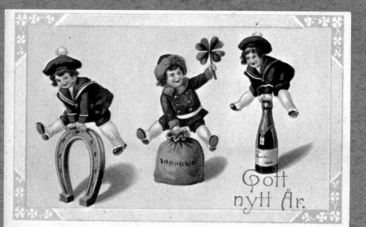

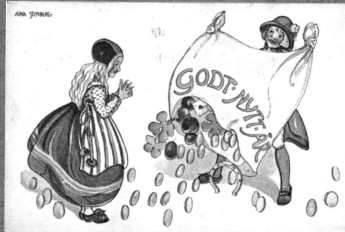

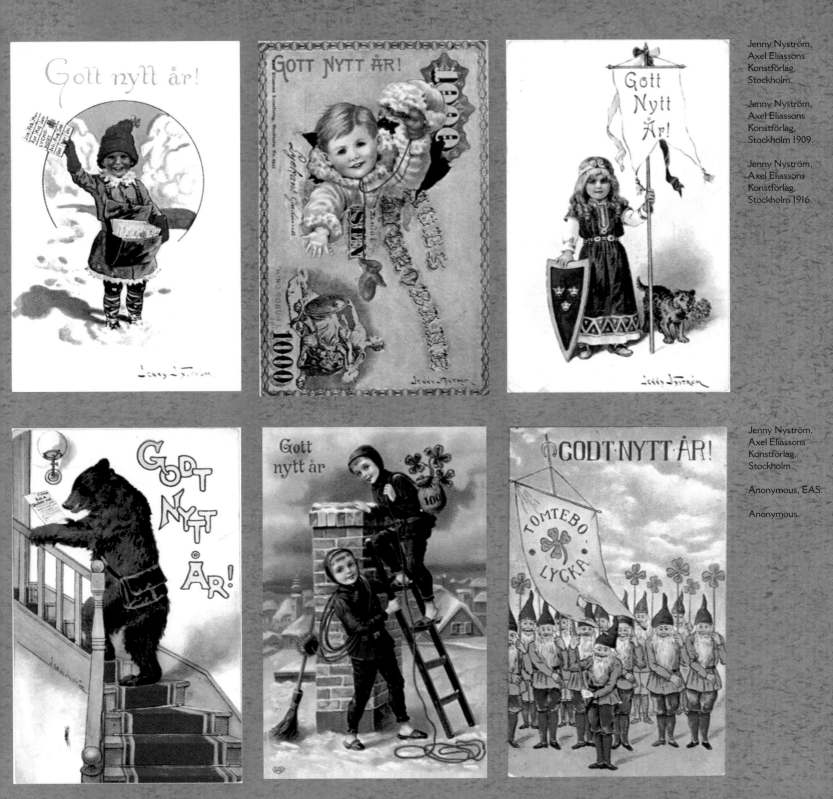

Jenny Nyström,
Axel Eliassons
Konstförlag,
Stockholm.

Jenny Nyström,
Axel Eliassons
Konstförlag,
Stockholm 1909.

Jenny Nyström,
Axel Eliassons
Konstförlag,
Stockholm 1916.

Jenny Nyström,
Axel Eliassons
Konstförlag,
Stockholm.

Anonymous, EAS.

Anonymous.

91

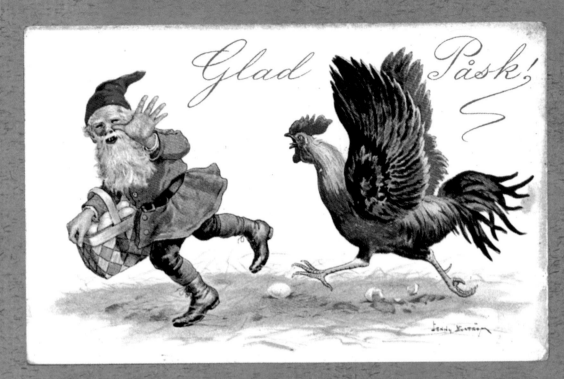

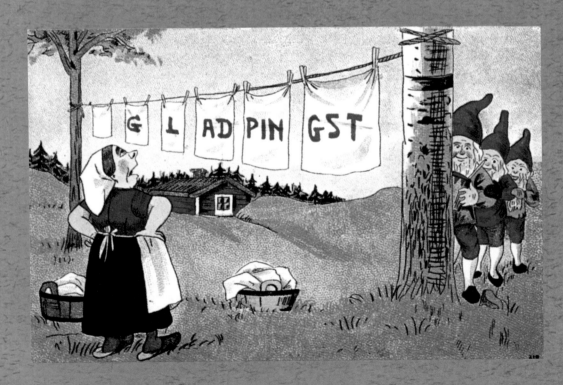

Postscript

Sources   Most of the cards are from Anna-Lisa Cederlund's huge collection. The Aina Stenberg cards were lent by her daughter Karin Jansson MasOlle. Other cards are from Postmuseum, Nordiska Museet, and the author's own collection. The text has been updated by the author for this English translation. Apart from interviews and newspaper articles, the following books have served as sources:

Ehrensvärd, Ulla **Den Svenska Tomten** (Svenska Turistföreningens förlag 1979)

Ehrensvärd, Ulla **Gamla Vykort** (Bonniers 1972)

Holt, Tonie and Valmai **Picture Postcards of the Golden Age** (MacvGibbon & Kee, London 1971)

Jäder, Karl och Astrid **Jenny Nyström** (Gummesons 1975)

Keyland, Nils **Julbröd, Julbockar och Staffanssång** (Svenska Teknologföreningens förlag 1919)

Liedholm, Alf **Julens ABC** (Forum 1971)

Nilsson, Martin **Festdagar och Vardagar** (Norstedts & Söners Förlag 1925)

Olsson, Marianne (Editor) **Julen För 100 År Sedan** (Tre Tryckare 1964)

Swahn, Jan-Öjvind **God Jul!** (Bonniers 1966)

Tillhagen, Carl-Herman (Editor) **Glada Juledagar** (Tre Tryckare 1965)

White, Gleeson **Christmas Cards and Their Chief Designers** (London 1895)

Collecting Christmas Cards

On December 23, 1939, an article in a Stockholm paper ended with the prophetic lines: "And we youngsters should perhaps consider collecting the Christmas cards of 1939. One day they will have a cultural value." The Christmas card is almost as old as the stamp and has now acquired a collector value. There are many devoted collectors in Sweden and abroad. Many Swedish cards fetch high prices at online and traditional auctions or at the specialized postcard antiquarians. Furthermore, Jenny Nyström's paintings as well as her Christmas card originals are highly coveted at auctions. This notwithstanding, the Christmas cards you received this year and the ones you may have kept are well worth a second look and perhaps even an album.

How to Date Cards

If it is hard to read the postmark on an older Swedish Christmas card, the back of the card can give you quite a bit of information. Until 1905, there was a designated space for name and address on the back of *Brefkortet* (see page 4). In 1900, the words *Carte Postale* were often added to *Brefkort*. After a spelling reform in 1906, most cards were spelled *Brevkort*. Between 1905 and 1910, *Brevkort* was sometimes translated into as many as 13 different languages. After 1910, there was just *Brevkort*, *Carte Postale*, or nothing at all. After 1930, there are sometimes series of numbers on the cards. The four numbers 3717, for example, tells you that the card was printed in 1937 and that the card was number 17 on the sheet. The number 225 on the other hand, shows a suggested retail price of SEK 2.25.

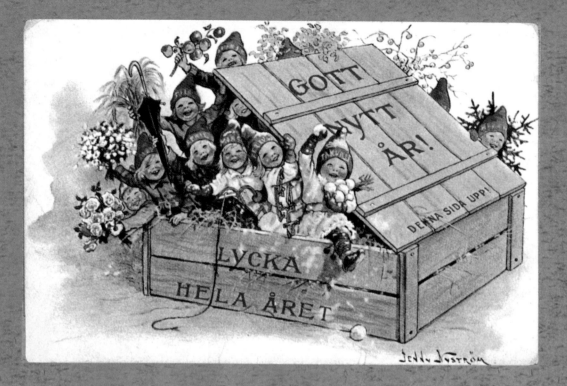

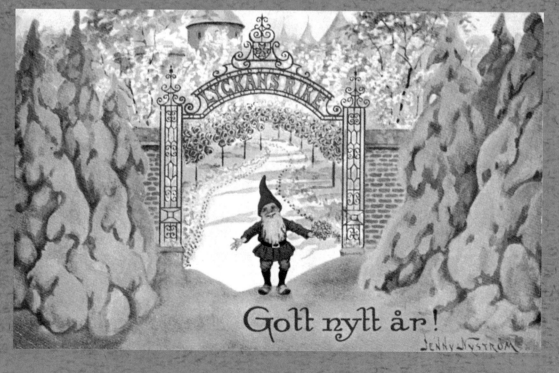

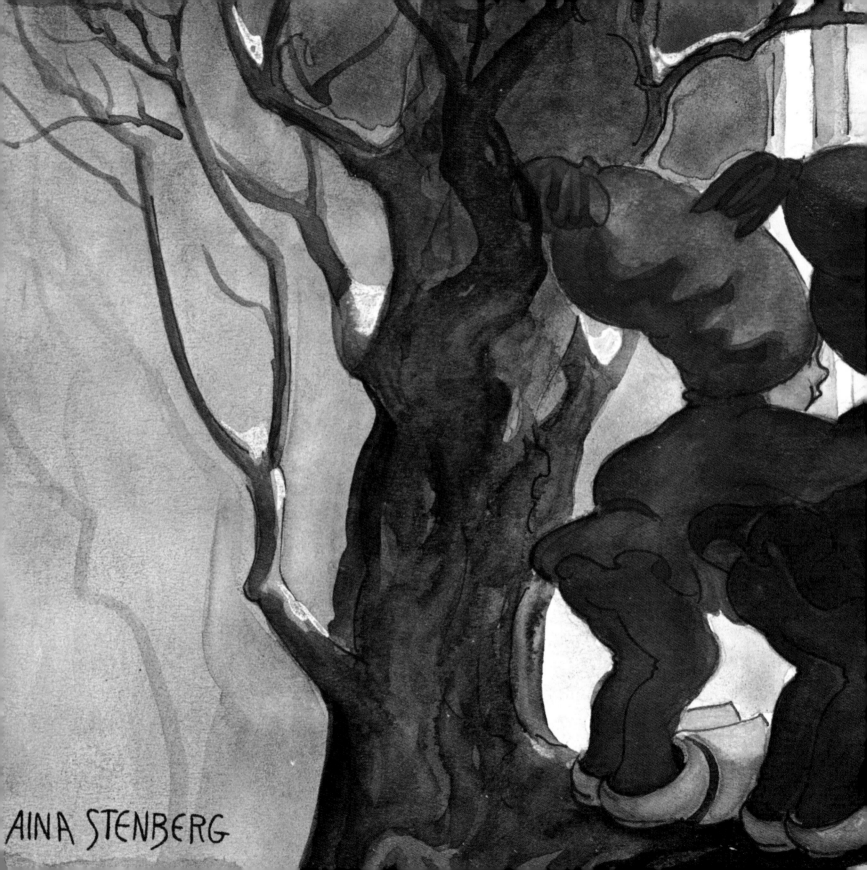

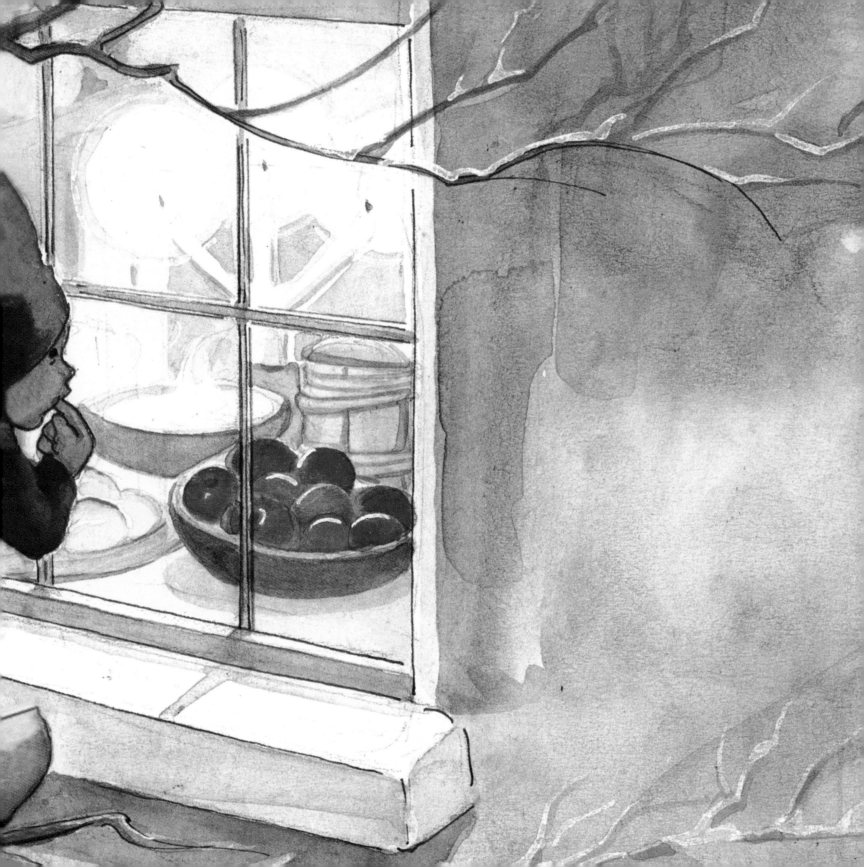